About the Author

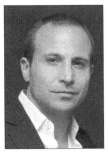

Dr. Joey Amato, DC, is a Principled Chiropractor who believes in body *maintenance* over body "treatment." By focusing on life, living, longevity, purpose, power, and action, he developed the Five Components to Absolute Emotional and Physical Health and lives them daily in his personal life and in his work promoting the tenets of principled health care.

A 2002 graduate of Life University in Marietta, Georgia, within a year Dr. Amato opened his first office, The Loft Chiropractic Life Center in New York City. In the ten years that followed, he gave presentations both locally and around the country, and added value to the lives of thousands of people with his seminars Raw Health, Survival of the Fittest, and The Gift. His clients range from infants and children, to everyday housewives and husbands, to professional athletes, actors, and performers, to top executives and CEOs.

"You are your #1 investment" is Dr. Amato's mantra. His single purpose in life is to assist people in understanding that the choices they make daily directly influence their emotional, physical, and financial health and stability. He works solely with those who understand their emotional and physical health is their own responsibility and who are willing to take direct charge of it so as to get more out of life.

Dr. Amato is CEO of Westchester Life Principled Healthcare and Pure Food and Drink body nourishment grab-and-go establishments. He wrote *The Absolute Truth & Common Sense!* to make his message of principled health care accessible to virtually anyone. An avid reader, Dr. Amato enjoys continuous learning from others who are successful and fulfilled in life, and knows that the readers of his book will be more informed and ready to take control of their own absolute emotional and physical health.

THE ABSOLUTE
TRUTH & COMMON SENSE!

THE ABSOLUTE
TRUTH & COMMON SENSE!

DR. JOEY AMATO

*For my children, Giuseppe Legend
and Viviana Love Amato*

Everything in life must have purpose, or else it is meaningless.

The purpose of this book is to *un*-educate you on old ways
of thinking, and *re*-educate you to think differently.
To change how you think, follow these recommendations:

EXPAND …	don't contract!
UPLIFT …	don't drag down!
USE POWER …	not force!
GIVE …	don't take!
SPEAK THE TRUTH …	not lies!
GIVE ASSURANCE …	not uncertainty!
SIMPLIFY …	don't complicate!
CLARIFY …	don't confuse!
ASK QUESTIONS …	get answers!
OPEN UP …	don't shut down!
THINK DIFFERENTLY …	not same old, same old!
CREATE LEADERS …	not followers!
CREATE HEROES …	not victims!
MAKE SENSE …	not hype!
BUILD RELATIONSHIPS …	don't break them!
GROW PROSPERITY …	not bankruptcy!
GO HIGHER …	not lower!
TAKE RESPONSIBILITY …	don't blame!
TAKE VICTORY …	over defeat!
SUCCEED …	don't fail!
BRING JOY …	not sorrow!

BUILD UP ...	don't destroy!
CREATE BALANCE ...	not imbalance!
ENHANCE LIFE ...	don't reduce it!
SUPPORT ...	don't interfere!
GET RESULTS ...	don't make excuses!
ADJUST ...	don't subluxate!
FULFILL ...	don't disappoint!
ALIGN ...	don't misalign!
THINK BIG ...	not little!
GIVE LOVE ...	not fear!
CONNECT ...	don't disconnect!
BE ACCOUNTABLE ...	not silent!
TAKE ACTION ...	don't wait!

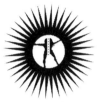

Table of Contents

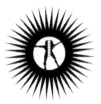

My Intention

My intention is to expand your present thought process, your present attitude, and your present belief system in regard to your emotional and physical health so that you can live in peace, love, and harmony, not only with your physical body but with everyone with whom you have contact. Please, for the time it takes to read this short book, let's play a game. I would like for you to use your imagination and pretend that everything you were taught has been erased from your present thought processes, attitudes, and belief systems. Imagine you are in a major science fiction motion picture or novel, and the knowledge of all the accumulated education you ever received from parents, grandparents, TV, teachers, preachers, doctors, psychiatrists, and institutions which manufacture and implement their ideas, theories, and guesses into society is no longer available for you to use to make decisions or identify with. Get the idea? Great! So we now have a pure, unadulterated, flexible, open mind with which to work, much like that of an infant: in other words, a clean slate!

Throughout, I will use the words *God, Universal Mind, Universal Intelligence, Universal Consciousness, Infinite Intelligence,* and *Creator* interchangeably, for this author understands these words to all mean the same great thing. Regardless of your religion or the rituals and customs you practice—or choose not to practice—we all, as human beings, can appreciate the observable fact that there is an Intelligence at work illuminating the cosmos, and thus creating life. This Intelligence can be observed in the world in which we live.

The foundation for emotional and physical health is based on simple concepts, facts, and universal truths.

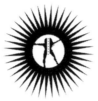

The Pure Principles

- God, the Creator, is universally intelligent!

- There is intelligence in the universe!

- This Universal Intelligence brings organization to all matter (objects) found in nature, thus maintaining it in existence for us, as human beings, to observe and identify with.

- This Universal Intelligence found in all natural matter continually gives to matter all its properties and actions, thus maintaining it in existence in the world in which we live.

- When this Universal Intelligence flows through living matter such as plants, animals, insects, and human beings, it is called *innate intelligence*. The flow of innate intelligence is normal.

- Innate intelligence creates, and is, life in living matter.

- There is nothing bigger than life itself!

- All living things have an innate, or inborn, wisdom that allows them to do what comes naturally (that is, innately) and normally. Plant roots know to grow down into the soil while the leaves grow up toward the sun; animals know how to give birth and feed their young;

insects know how to search for nourishment and reproduce. This is nature. We appreciate this innate intelligence and call it instinct. All these living creatures know what to do instinctively (that is, innately) and are healthy if they are left alone in their natural, normal state.

- Health is the normal expression of the innate intelligence in a living organism. Health exists as long as nothing interferes with the process of that expression.

- Interference with the connection of the innate intelligence in a living organism results in a decrease in that organism's innate intelligence, which deteriorates life within that organism, making it susceptible to long-term sickness, disease, deterioration, degeneration, physical deformity, and premature death. These are the negative effects that result from interference.

- Human beings are a part of this universe. As such, they and all living organisms are subject to these universal laws.

- Human beings also have an inborn, innate intelligence that is both observable and identifiable. Examples include conception and giving birth—acts which, for centuries, have required no assistance. Nature simply ran its course instinctively and normally. Other examples include an infant's ability to naturally and instinctively roll over onto his or her belly, lift their head to see, begin the process of crawling, and then eventually walking. No human being is responsible for educating an infant in this process; these acts come naturally, instinctively, and innately, for the infant possesses the innate intelligence that expresses life.

- No human being's conscious thinking is responsible for the countless number of cellular activities that take place daily for body maintenance or for adapting to internal and external environments with activities such as respiration, digestion, waste removal, body temperature regulation, hormone regulation, etc. This is all done innately (that is, automatically). It just is!

- It is not complicated to understand these natural universal laws, which *are*, *have always been*, and *will always be* a normal part of all living organisms.

> These principles are time-tested, absolute truths
> that make sense and never need to be defended.
> They can, however, be observed and discussed!

Remember our game: This is the only information you were ever taught to identify with regarding your emotional and physical stability—this information is what creates your thought process, attitude, and belief system for the present and for the future, and directly impacts the quality of your life.

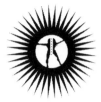

Your Life Is a Gift!

From the information previously provided, it would make logical sense that God, the Universal Intelligence, created us to be emotionally and physically healthy. The life we all have is a normal part of nature requiring nothing more than a conscious effort and physical application to support that life by doing everything in our power to avoid interference with the natural processes of life. As you read on, those things that interfere with the natural, normal state of life will become apparent, as will how this interference not only negatively affects your own emotional, physical, and financial health, but also the lives of everyone else with whom you come into contact. This is the law of cause and effect. Understanding and appreciating this law is truly a gift. Use your free will wisely, for it is what separates us from all other living creatures and makes us each so special and unique.

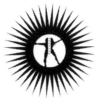

Being Pure Principled:
The Definition of Health

Emotional and physical health is the ability to function normally: physically, mentally, emotionally, socially, and spiritually without long-term sickness and debilitating diseases. Emotional and physical health results in a quality of life that allows you to give love and receive love; to give joy and receive joy; and to feel fulfilled by having the ability to achieve and appreciate whatever your own personal goals may be.

Repetition is the mother of skill!
It's not enough to hear or read it once!

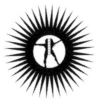

Chapter 1

Knowing the Difference: Common Sense through Observance

"Just because emotional and physical disease is so common in America, does not make it normal!" —Dr. Joey Amato, DC

"Is it better to know one thing that works than a million things that aren't so and don't work!" —Dr. B. J. Palmer, DC

"Man has freedom of choice, without which there would be no accountability or responsibility!" —Dr. David R. Hawkins, MD, PhD

Every product has a producer. Nine out of ten human-made products come with an instruction manual. Instruction manuals are typically for the operation and/or assembly of a product. The manual shows you, the consumer, how to properly assemble and operate your newly purchased product, ensuring you will get the maximum enjoyment, benefit, and lifespan from it. Instruction manuals exist for only human-made products; manuals are neither seen nor found in nature. Through humankind's observance of nature, humans have developed theories, guesses, and opinions that are then used to educate other humans on what is *believed* to be true at the time. It's both funny and disturbing when you realize the number of times over the centuries humans have postulated, guessed, and theorized about an idea that was accepted, only to be proven wrong years later. It is equally true that many great men and women have been put to death for saying things considered against the grain of established thought of the time, only to be proven true many years later. Undoubtedly, humankind has had, and still does have, moments of clarity and ignorance that can be easily recognized by using good old common sense. Just observe the natural order that balances the universe. The universe and that which resides in it, such as nature, is *always* balancing itself. The universe always knows what to do, when to do it, how to do it, and what amounts to do it in—all the time.

Is it wise to have more faith in humans who are prone to make mistakes than in the Intelligence that created the universe and life? Why do human beings not come with an instruction manual on how to properly operate their own emotional and physical systems? The answer is simple: common sense. The fact is, we are more than just a body that is broken down into systems and parts similar to the products we invent. Humans have taken something *so simple* and made it complex; we have divided up the body and taught that it operates like the parts of a machine. There is nothing wrong with humankind's quest to understand him- or herself as long as there is common sense and logic working with our ability to observe the Intelligence that exists all around us. The problem occurs when Man's guesses and theories are accepted as facts, then instructed and marketed to the population, and later become institutionalized into the fabric of society. It is equally disturbing that this is done under the illusion of serving humankind when it is obvious that most of the time it hurts us emotionally, physically, and financially.

We can see these side effects easily within the failure of our own American allopathic medical system. At present, America is the *unhealthiest* country in the world. We have been trained to focus on sickness, disease, deterioration, degeneration, deformity, death, medical necessity, diagnosis, and treatment protocols, rather than on *life, living, longevity, purpose, power* and *action*. We are the unhealthiest country because we treat diagnoses and symptoms and do not remove the interferences that prevent the body from healing naturally. In fact, our present system directly interferes with the body's ability to heal itself intelligently. The reason humans do not come with an instruction manual is because we are given everything needed to innately *sustain* our quality of life.

We have to first observe our environment and then ask the right questions. A great first question is: Are we human beings or are we just assembled body parts? If we are, in fact, human beings, then what is a human being? I daresay a human being is a soul, a mind, and a physical body. I also daresay our individual soul is our innate, inward intelligence connected to God—the Universal Intelligence—which gave, and continues to give, life, and is life. There is nothing bigger than life! We use our mind to interpret what we observe and experience inwardly and outwardly with our internal and external senses, so we can then, by choice, express creatively what we have comprehended and perceived. This is *thinking* and this creates our thoughts and beliefs from our environment. As a result, from our thoughts we can physically act from this connection out of gratitude that inspires us to inspire others.

Everything begins with a thought, and that fact gives us the power to create or destroy. Long before the first brick was laid down to build the Empire State Building someone had an inspired, creative thought. This connection to God, the Universal Mind, or whatever you wish to call this connection that inspires, is referred to as *being graced*. This connection to Infinite Intelligence is what fills our hearts and brings us feelings of joy. In fact, this is love, and love inspires purpose that leads us to greatness.

Fear, on the other hand, cripples us first emotionally and then physically if we do not understand and utilize it correctly. The true feeling of joy comes from our purpose to serve humankind and it is selfless; it asks nothing in return and yet always gives back in great abundance. Our physical bodies are the vehicles through which we act to experience this union of soul, mind, and physical body. This great connection expands, creates, and heals. In contrast, fear contracts, destroys, and brings about emotional and physical sickness, disease, deterioration, degeneration, deformity, and premature death. If misunderstood and uncorrected, fear will always negatively affect a human beings' quality of life. The universe gives the human physical body everything to nourish its soul and mind, and nature gives the body everything needed to nourish its mind and physical body. Some of the most important names in history all understood and used these principles.

Anything that interferes with a person's soul, mind, and physical body's connection will result in disease and chaos, and cause disharmony that will bring about sickness, disease, deterioration, degeneration, deformity, and premature death. We can observe this in how Americans currently regard emotional and physical health: We treat diagnoses and labels; we do not *maintain* human beings. No matter the circumstances, you can always realign your own thinking by observing. Use common sense and reestablish this emotional, mental connection. I call this *knowing the difference* and this is the first factor of the first component to emotional and physical health.

What matters in life is how you perceive circumstances, how you determine decisions, and how you physically act upon them. Your choices are always yours to make and it is your responsibility to yourself as well as to your offspring and those who rely upon you, to *know the difference*. The choices you make determine your emotional and physical health. For children it's not that simple, however; they do what they are told based on their parents' interpretation of the world and how they choose to perceive it. Parents need to know the truth and take back full responsibility for their children's lives. Simply put, you either want *more* or you want less; you are either *connected* or disconnected; *aligned* or misaligned; *growing* or shrinking; *flexible* or inflexible; or *moving toward health* or toward sickness, disease, deterioration, degeneration, deformity, and premature death.

What is your #1 asset? Could it be you? The Pure Principles presented in the following pages support life, living, longevity, purpose, power, and action in a practical, applicable manner. It is just common sense through our observance of the universe and nature, which is a tremendous part of our environment. Although we did not need an instruction manual in the beginning, it seems we definitely need one now. Follow your heart and start *supporting* life! The quality of your life and of those who rely on you requires you to make the right choices. Invest in what matters. Invest in yourself and your family. Share your life and its purpose with others on a daily basis and watch your relationships grow. This will have a positive impact for you at home, at work, and personally. It's no secret; it's common sense! Either do what you love or love what you do, but always know your personal power. The choice is yours; you have that something called *free will*, which is what makes us human beings. One seed planted in the soil and given the right conditions will bring forth many, many more seeds. This is God's multiplication! It is not complex and we do not need to fully understand it, for we can easily see the benefits in its simplicity. Observe it and use it daily to create emotional and physical health in yourself and in those who rely on you. That which supports life is supported by life. Your thoughts and beliefs control your actions. *Know the difference* and *take action* now!

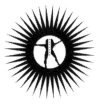

Chapter 2

The Genius Within Inspires Purpose and Power

"Right now billions of billions of trillions of trillions of functions are happening in your body that mere man cannot comprehend!"
—Dr. Joey Amato, DC

"What is the value of education if it fails?" —Dr. B. J. Palmer, DC

"Human history is the record of man's struggle to comprehend truths which to those of genius appear obvious." —Dr. David R. Hawkins, MD, PhD

What are the right conditions for emotional and physical health? We know that some seeds take root, sprout, and flourish to produce many more seeds, while other seeds never take root. Perhaps by observing our natural environment and the world around us, we will learn yet another life lesson. I am of the absolute belief we all are born with specific, innate qualities which I will refer to as the *Genius Within*. This inner genius is the source of our attributes and talents which are a direct result of the connection we have to the Intelligence in the universe that most human beings refer to as God. Do not confuse Genius Within with intelligence quotient (IQ). Our IQ comes from *outside* (external) education and is the recognition and comprehension of symbols and words, whereas the Genius Within is the *inner* voice that inspires us emotionally to be creative. That inspiration gives birth to our purpose to live and allows our creative self to be expressed through physical actions which consequently give life to our personal power. This gives us joy and allows us to receive joy that leads to fulfillment. Our inner genius and outside-educated IQ can work together in harmony, and, when they do, it is always reflected in our emotional and physical health. This is the foundation that creates a stable, lasting purpose.

One seed planted under the right conditions brings about many more seeds, making its purpose of life everlasting. You do not give a man a fish; rather, you teach him how to fish so he never goes hungry. This is everlasting! It takes nothing for a single, lit candle to light a thousand candles, so that no one ever has to be without light. This is everlasting! What does it take to give a smile, a friendly gesture, or a word of encouragement to a stranger, a friend, or a family member, while asking nothing in return? It *takes nothing* but it always *gives something*, and ironically this act usually gives more to the one giving than to the one receiving. If you ask nothing and expect nothing in return, you will never be disappointed, regardless of how others respond. These acts reinforce your inner genius and allow you to go from a lower to higher level of consciousness, to *open your mind* and change your present thought process, attitude, and belief system. This ensures your constant *growth* and *progression* forward, not backward, all of which supports emotional and physical health.

When you understand this, you create and develop your personal purpose and your personal power. Never give your personal power away through fear to someone you consider, at that moment, to be in a greater position of authority. When you give your personal power away, you allow someone else to dictate what is best for you. Free will allows you to use your common sense through observance, to have both positive and negative experiences in order to grow, and over time, to create wisdom. When you appreciate this in life, you are emotionally happier because you are *in control,* which creates the chemistry needed for emotional and physical health. Your inner potential, your Genius Within, is then ready for circumstances and opportunities that would otherwise be overlooked and unrecognized. If feelings of self-doubt, negative emotions, or an overblown ego interfere with your connection to your inner genius, you miss many opportunities to elevate your personal success, and thereby negatively affect your emotional and physical health.

If utilized properly, however, self-doubt, negative emotions, and the ego can work with your inner genius as a compass to guide you when you are temporarily lost. This is where *knowing the difference* comes into play; by recognizing these feelings and accepting them as a normal part of your consciousness, you are allowed to ask yourself quality questions and receive quality answers to enlighten and then inspire you. These moments of inspiration come as a direct result of feeling grateful for being connected to something of a higher nature. Acknowledging the Genius Within inspires and gives ideas that will always illuminate your way from a lesser level of creativity to a higher one. When you appreciate and are grateful for both the obstacles and the rewards in your life, you also recognize the Genius Within. When you are grateful for experiences, whether they are good or bad, you are elevated and graced with inspiration. We commonly refer to this inner knowledge as a *gut feeling,* the *voice within,* or the *inner voice,* and, when we act on it, it is always followed by positive results. When you take the time to recognize *knowing the difference,* you truly appreciate the lessons learned and *take full responsibility* for your actions.

When you take responsibility, you eliminate blame—something which, over time, cripples you emotionally and physically. This knowledge and its application are what create wisdom. We need both positive and negative experiences to constantly elevate us to higher levels of fulfillment and personal success. This is something that money cannot, and will never be able to, replace unless you receive the money for services you render that benefit humankind emotionally and physically.

Many corporations and consumers fail to recognize this important universal fact. The fact that million-dollar marketing campaigns sell tons of products to consumers does not mean the products sold necessarily support long-term emotional and physical health. Take the processed fast-food industry as an example. The feel-good feelings many associate with these types of products are temporary and short-lived, which creates an immediate demand for more. Material items do not provide long-term peace, love, or inner harmony—those intangibles I will refer to as *inner joy* and *fulfillment*. It is akin to trying to live a healthy lifestyle by eating processed, synthetic, human-made "foods"; they never nourish your physical body, so you eat and eat and need to eat more because the cells in your body crave nourishment. Under these conditions, they actually lack nourishment and this creates the need for more. Again, common sense and *knowing the difference* make you aware that money and products you purchase are simply tools you can utilize as you endeavor to live a life that supports emotional and physical health.

Always invest in yourself, for you are your #1 asset. Recognizing this potential within yourself makes all the difference in your quality of life now and during your later years. How you live your life emotionally and physically will be respected and honored long after your death, and the legacy you leave behind will make all the difference for future generations to emulate. Leaving behind only material wealth is not enough, as it cannot be enjoyed if the people you leave it to lack emotional and physical health.

The principles discussed in this short book are everlasting. The principles you live by and your personal purpose will be carried forward by the people in those relationships you have created. Nurture the Genius Within and know your purpose and your personal power, for they work with whichever resources you make available to them. The Universal Mind, that Universal Intelligence, knows more than educated humans. Do you have more faith in what humans produce than in what has created and expands the cosmos, grows a tree, or reproduces billions of living organisms daily? Observe the natural world around you and begin to appreciate it, for you are a part of it and not above its laws. Relinquish old ways and bad habits that no longer serve you so as to always ensure growth in a positive direction. Stay connected to life's genius! Be flexible, adjust, realign, and get connected emotionally and physically. *Your thoughts and beliefs control your actions!* Either you are growing, or you are shrinking. And if you are shrinking, you are prematurely dying!

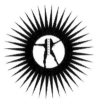

Chapter 3

Flexibility: Adapting to Change

*"Surrender your old ways for new ways and start anew as winter ends
and spring begins. The cycle of life's purpose is everlasting!"*
—Dr. Joey Amato, DC

*"Usually the second wave of disappointments comes because you never
dealt with the first ones!"* —Dr. Sid E. Williams, DC

At times we find it difficult to keep pace with the rapidly changing world in which we live. The amount of information and the speed with which it is delivered is overwhelming and causes much confusion. If confusion is not understood for what it really is, it leads to frustration; mounting frustration leads to worry; and worry leads to negative thoughts and beliefs that are reinforced daily in our own minds by the words we use internally and externally. This results in negative thought processes, attitudes, and belief systems which affect our emotional and physical health and breed negative habits. This is then reflected in how we perceive and speak about the world. We can instantly grow to a higher level of consciousness if we *know the difference* and use common sense to logically reinforce with absolute authority the ability to accept things beyond our immediate control and relinquish what is of no long-term benefit to us. This is what matters daily. This generates self-satisfaction with long-term benefits that serve you and all others with whom you come into contact. When we relinquish negative thoughts, we immediately breathe a sigh of relief as the pressure is lifted and we are able to realign ourselves. This puts us back in emotional alignment with the Infinite Intelligence and reestablishes balance and order.

In nature, through observation, common sense, and logic, we easily note the change of seasons that occurs naturally around the world. Living organisms such as insects, animals, and plants have to adapt or die. It is that simple: adapt or die. So, in certain parts of the world when summer ends and fall begins, the living organisms that live in these locations have to accept the change that winter is coming. If those living organisms do not adapt to change by accepting the reality of winter, they will die off and suffer extinction. In winter, in certain parts of the world, it is evident that a drastic change occurs and this natural process is normal. When spring returns, it brings forth regrowth and new life. Nature and everything in it—except that which is blessed with free will—understands this natural phenomenon inherently, for it is connected to the intelligence that flows within it, which is its life. All living organisms have to adapt or die. This is true. But how we die is our choice.

We, on the other hand, have been given the gift of free will and, though the same universal laws apply to us, we struggle with our emotional and physical health and the ability to adapt and get stronger physically as we age. We, too, expand and contract emotionally and physically, like the change of seasons, and have great potential, but our environment easily influences our thoughts. What influences us as a society? What influences you as an individual? If, in fact, we are part of this Universal Consciousness, and if the same universal laws apply to us, as does everything in our observable environment (that is, nature), why are so many infants, children, adolescents, adults, and elderly emotionally and physically sick, diseased, deteriorated, degenerated, deformed, and dying prematurely? Of particular note, in America these numbers grow astronomically year after year. Common sense dictates that this is more than mere coincidence, or it is what the media sells in order to influence our thoughts and beliefs.

Another important question the average American citizen does not ask is: Why do all the sickness, disease, deterioration, degeneration, deformity, and premature deaths occur only in America in the excessive numbers that are recorded yearly? The numbers are, in fact, not the same around the world, as our media would lead us to believe. The numbers have steadily climbed in America since the 1800s. Is this normal or natural? No one person can distort the facts.

Presently America represents only about 5% of the total world population, but we are ranked first in terms of the number of incidents of every disease known to humankind. Also disturbing is the fact that America has the highest number of diseases ever recorded since its discovery. According to recent studies America ranks #1 in the following:

- infants dying before and after childbirth;
- autism;
- all types of surgeries;
- cancer;
- heart disease, degenerative diseases, autoimmune disorders, neuro-logical dysfunctions, stomach irritations, childhood disabilities,

childhood cancers, and emotional disorders such as depression and anxiety and others too numerous to list;

- obesity, physical deformity, and the largest number of people requiring assistance with canes, walkers, wheelchairs, bedside assistance, visiting nurses, and home care attendants, as well as the use of scooters and other mobile devices for people who have become legally disabled and handicapped;

- the number of people institutionalized in mental health facilities receiving legalized, FDA-approved medications and treatment protocols such as electroshock therapy (treatments such as these still go on in mental institutions for what has been labeled "chemical imbalances" in the brain);

- teenagers on legalized, FDA-approved medications;

- teenagers committing suicide;

- people being incarcerated in the U.S. penal system; and

- the use of legalized, FDA-approved medications for emotional and physical disabilities.

The people of the United States are, without a doubt, the undisputed champions in the world when it comes to emotional and physical sickness, disease, deterioration, degeneration, deformity, and premature death. I challenge you to ask *why?* Again, I simply ask why are we the only country suffering with such heavy burdens? Does God, who is the Universal Intelligence, the Universal Consciousness, and our Creator, just not like America, Americans, or any first-generation immigrants and their offspring? This question is reasonable given that #1) I have children and #2) I live here! Clearly, America has a problem and/or situation that does not seem to be getting resolved with our current level of thinking. Maybe it is time to change that current level of thinking. Wouldn't you agree?

America has the largest and most profitable corporations in the world financing the most "research" ever conducted in the history of humankind on every psychiatrist-labeled "mental disorder" there is. These labels are documented in the Diagnostic and Statistical Manual of Mental Disorders (DSM), the psychiatrists' bible. Year after year this book gets thicker and thicker. Likewise, these large and profitable corporations finance the most "research" on every labeled "physical disorder" documented in the Physician's Desk Reference (PDR), the allopathic medical doctors' bible. It, too, continues to expand year after year—much like the waistlines of our population.

This expansion of labels commonly referred to as *diagnoses* is not only growing, but is also what directly influences what Americans call *health care*. Is this "health care"? Are people "healthier"? Are our children "healthier"? This daily marketing of influential rhetoric is now our current level of consciousness, and has been for some time. Quite simply, Americans have been trained to believe in sickness, disease, deterioration, degeneration, deformity, and premature death, and accept them as normal parts of their lives. Once people are labeled, they are placed on "treatment" protocols that never end, are costly, and always produce side effects. Americans have been trained to view their bodies as though they are just a collection of body parts. That is the mental disconnection that affects people first emotionally then physically. Readjust your thoughts, get aligned, be flexible, and get connected! You are a human being, not a victim. Your thoughts and beliefs control your actions. To paraphrase from the Bible, know the truth and it shall set you free, first emotionally, then physically. If you think, believe, and act like a victim, then you *are* a victim and you render yourself powerless. Use your common sense and observe your environment; let the Genius Within express love and appreciation for this new level of consciousness. Your health is your responsibility; it is a personal matter between *you* and *yourself*, no matter how many people you let get involved. That is your personal power!

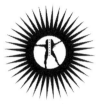

Chapter 4

Power of Words: The Language Used Determines the Path Followed

"In 'health care' facts are facts, truth is truth, nature is nature, common sense is common sense, and lies are lies, and the responsibility to ourselves comes from and is spoken to ourselves through words; it is as simple as that!" —Dr. Joey Amato, DC

"Medical doctors work toward a standard of health care in which they and the drug companies think they know!" —Dr. B. J. Palmer, DC

"Apparently, from untold millions of individual experiences in one's life, usually only a few lessons are ever learned." —Dr. David R. Hawkins, MD, PhD

"Until your thought is changed, your conditions never will be, your body never will be." —Ernest Holmes (1887-1960)

"The greatest discovery of any generation is that human beings can alter their lives by altering the attitudes of their minds." —Albert Schweitzer (1875-1965)

Consider these two questions: What seeds are you planting in your thoughts? Are you creating the right conditions? Given the right conditions a seed has one combined purpose: to take root, sprout, produce more seeds, and continue the cycle of life. A seed does not have decision-making powers since it has a single objective: multiply in great abundance and supply, and thrive and adapt to fulfill its purpose of life. Its responsibility is inherent in its innate intelligence to do what it knows to do, and nothing more than that.

Human beings, on the other hand, possess emotional minds and the power to decide from choices that come from their thoughts. Your thought processes, attitudes, and belief systems are in your emotional mind; when you use your mind to think, you use words to comprehend meaning. Thinking is nothing more than the use of words to ask and answer questions that creates feelings. Feelings are emotions that give us the fuel needed to pursue our goals, whatever they may be. I daresay that the answers you receive from thinking come from either the accumulated experiences which have created your present belief system, the Genius Within, or both.

Our connection to our inner genius inspires and connects us to a higher nature that always serves us first so that we are ready and capable to serve humankind. When you *know the difference*, you can work with experience, education, and the inner genius simultaneously to receive answers that will bring about higher thoughts of consciousness to create personal joy and fulfillment. This creates your purpose in life. You can only receive inspiration when you choose to be grateful and appreciative for your life and life experiences, whether they are positive or negative. So when you think in this way, it is nothing more than asking and answering specific questions, and you will only be as great as the quality of words chosen for the questions you seek to have answered.

What we as human beings use to interpret and explain the meanings of things are words. Words are very powerful and can be used for good or bad depending on the intentions of the user. Proverbs 18:20 states, "Death and life are in the power of the tongue, and they that love it shall eat the fruit thereof." Simply put, words are the seeds of human thought which creates our thought processes, attitudes, and belief systems, and thus our perception of the world around us. As adults it is our responsibility to provide the right conditions to ensure the absolute best emotional, physical, and financial health for our families, communities, and ourselves. Depending on how words are interpreted, they are powerful enough to elicit chemical discharges (nerve impulses, hormones, etc.). Our bodies physically react through the nervous system in either a positive, beneficial manner that builds us up or in a negative, destructive manner that breaks us down. Consider someone who is diagnosed (labeled) with a disease. The individual that is diagnosed feels fear from the words used because their very meaning elicits a negative emotional response that leads to a negative physical response. Certain words are good and certain words are bad. Certain words empower and certain words render us powerless. This is a perfect example of the universal law of cause and effect.

All universal laws are absolute and when not used correctly manifest dire consequences that, over time, always result in emotional and physical instability. When you violate a universal law that governs and balances the universe, nature, and everything in it, you become out of alignment, off balance, and disconnected. It does not matter whether the law is broken by intention or by accident; a universal law is law, and it is impersonal to circumstances or events. When laws are broken, symptoms and situations such as emotional distress, physical fatigue, pain, organ discomfort, and many other symptoms develop—all situations that require our immediate attention. When we blame symptoms that occur in our bodies on some enemy outside the body or on some malfunctioning body part, we simply demonstrate how misinformed we are. Also, we were neither taught nor reinforced with the difference between being connected and disconnected, balanced and out of balance, aligned and misaligned, or flexible and inflexible.

The words I choose to use, such as *blame, enemy from outside the body*, and *malfunctioning body part*, are words upon which I, too, was raised through the media and pharmaceutical corporate influence. These words influenced my parents and all those around me. I was raised with a medicine chest that was secretly and conveniently stashed behind the bathroom mirror in my childhood home. I was raised to blame some outside, invisible "enemy" every time I had a sniffle, stuffy nose, cough, body ache, chill, or any other physical complaint. There was always some magical, legalized, FDA-approved pharmaceutical drug, pill, or liquid that would ease my symptoms and defeat that nasty germ, bacteria, virus, or whatever the enemy was called at that time. My body had no say in the matter or the process, and supposedly was just as helpless as I.

These legal drugs were missing from my body chemistry because the Universe did not properly place them there when I was created. These drugs were needed in order to reestablish my health. In effect, I was defective from conception to birth. Since I was defective, I did not have everything I needed to sustain life, or so my parents and I were first told, and then sold. This is what was taught, marketed, and reinforced through specifically chosen words—words that were fed to my parents and their parents, and then taught to me, thereby creating a thought process, family attitude, and family belief system for our family's emotional and physical health. Because they had been trained to do so, my parents gave their authority over their children to the family allopathic medical doctor, someone they barely knew in life.

In fact, in all my experiences growing up, I was never once taught the truth: that germs and bacteria are necessary scavengers that clean up dead and dying cellular debris resulting from cells dying and new cells replacing the dead ones. I was not taught that this is a normal part of the process of life. I was not taught that human beings and every other living organism are all self-sustaining and that each plays a role in the ecosystem and balance of nature. In fact, my family and I were taught just the opposite. Only as I grew older and began to take responsibility for my own thoughts and actions did I empower myself with the use of my own common sense through observance.

Through experience I developed my personal power to think logically and question everything concerning my emotional and physical health. I soon realized that germs, bacteria, microbes, or whatever other names the drug corporation scientists wanted to call those things, are actually necessary parts of life. Simply put, without germs and bacteria we would not be here. Why do germs proliferate so rapidly when we are sick, diseased, deteriorating, degenerating, deforming, and dying prematurely? Because that is what they do. They eat stuff that is dying. If a *part* of you is dying prematurely, then *you* are dying prematurely and these tiny microbes will bring you back to the earth and recycle you.

This law of cause-and-effect is present in every aspect of our emotional and physical health because it is law. For every effect there is a cause; in the case of a human body overridden with germs, bacteria, or whatever label is used, the cause is due to the interference of normal nerve transmission. If the nerve cannot send its signals to organ systems the way it is intended, the physical body's resistance is lowered and cells die prematurely creating dis-ease. Dis-ease leads to disease, deterioration, degeneration, deformity, and diagnosis—which all lead to allopathic medical treatment protocols with harsh legal drugs and surgeries with harsh side effects. This "treatment," in fact, creates more interference to nerve transmission. Any interference of the life force that decreases normal nerve transmission will result in germs and bacteria being signaled to clean up the dying tissue cells. As our physical body deteriorates over time, the germs and bacteria multiply faster, and create what is commonly referred to as an infection, which, in our society, leads to more allopathic medical treatments.

Many things cause interference to normal nerve transmissions, for example: physical trauma; repetitive work and lifestyle habits; man-made chemicals found in what is sold as "food"; cleaning products; all legalized, FDA-approved pharmaceutical drugs; and the list—in America—goes on and on. Consider this: If an organ is slowly decaying, the normal course is for a germ and bacteria to eat it. Why? Because everything in the universe has been created to maintain balance and order. We are made from elements from the earth and the earth is made of elements from space. When we die, we return to the earth, thanks to tiny microbes—microbes the media demonize to help sell all those legal, FDA-approved drugs. Universal Intelligence created everything to always be balanced. A seed cannot take root or sprout if the conditions are not right. Germs and bacteria are always present in the body; every one of us has every germ and bacteria the nightly news reports talk about, with the exception of some human-made, factory-farmed bacteria that can be easily avoided.

The media spreads fear with scary words, telling us we might catch "it." For well over 90% of the time, this simply is not true, and for the other less-than-10% of the time, it is due to the negligence of the processed, multi-trillion-dollar-a-year, human-made food industry. Every human being lives symbiotically with microbes we call germs and bacteria; on a cellular level, they are the house cleaners of our bodies' deepest areas. This is fact, not opinion; it can be easily verified if you take responsibility for your own health.

Antoine Béchamp, French chemist and biologist, was one of the first to recognize this. He stated, "Whenever there is anything in nature that is dying, or beginning to decay, something comes and eats it up." This is nature's way of cleaning up dead tissue cells and eliminating them as waste. The human body gets rid of waste by way of exhalation of carbon dioxide, removal of fecal matter, urine, sweat, and by germs and bacteria. When you are run down emotionally and choose to live in fear of sickness, disease, deterioration, degeneration, deformity, premature death, germs, bacteria, viruses, and anything else the media and pharmaceutical industrial complex is selling this week, then your own physical body will react to this way of thinking by creating an attitude and belief system which creates the wrong conditions and results in physical negative effects. When you are placed on legal, FDA-approved drugs for your symptoms or blood test results, you are simply subluxating the nervous system's ability to heal. This prolongs the symptoms and causes what is believed to be a need for even more legal, FDA-approved drugs. When this is consistently repeated over the years, it manifests the wrong environment and leads to long-term sickness, disease, deterioration, degeneration, deformity, and premature death. This affects your #1 investment: you!

Interference with the nervous system affects our quality of life, which affects relationships and the ability to enjoy the fruits of our labor. A perfect example of interfering with the nervous system is when you have a headache. There must be a cause that creates the headache, but most Americans have been trained to take over-the-counter, legalized, FDA-approved medications called *nostrums*. These legalized, FDA-approved medications paralyze (interfere with) the central nervous system's ability to feel the headache, which paralyzes its ability to send signals to your mind, thus disabling your ability to receive the alarm that something is wrong. It has been documented that prolonged use of legal, FDA-approved headache medications leads to internal hemorrhaging and then to what we know as a stroke or aneurysm. Most legal, FDA-approved drugs "treat" only the symptoms and not the cause, but they all produce more symptoms and more sickness with prolonged use. Think of it this way: If your child's school was on fire and the principal shut off the alarm that would normally alert the fire department, what would happen to the children? Get the point? Symptoms are great, for they tell you that you need to get aligned and connected by removing the interference(s) that causes something called *subluxations*.

Subluxations that go unchecked and uncorrected destroy our emotional and physical health. Just as the body needs germs and bacteria to make it stronger, the body also needs symptoms and situations to tell us when we are disconnected in some way so that we can get reconnected and balance the system as a whole. The idea that germs, bacteria, or whatever threat is being sold this week might cause sickness, disease, deterioration, degeneration, deformity, and premature death is false. When you use common sense through observation and take responsibility for questioning everything, you easily recognize how true this is. Subluxations occur first, and cause dysfunction in muscles, joints, tendons, ligaments, and connective tissue, which then manifests into symptoms. Repetitive negative emotional thoughts, accidental physical trauma, lifestyle repetitive physical habits, and man-made toxins in the food supply along with numerous other man-made toxins found in many products all cause severe subluxations.

The idea that your genes cause sickness, disease, deterioration, degeneration, deformity, and premature death is as ridiculous as the idea that germs and bacteria do the same. Once again, if you believe this, the responsibility is taken off your shoulders and placed in the hands of someone you allow to have authority over you. Your personal power can be taken away when the wrong word or words elicit fear. The wrong word for you is the right word for business. I know I was created, and that which created me and gave me life and free will did not do this so that I could relinquish my responsibility to myself and give it to someone else out of fear. Get rid of the false habits and thoughts that have been engrained into your mind from childhood. These thoughts of blame reduce your strength and will be the chains that hold you back from higher levels of consciousness that always bring peace, love, and happiness, and that create a joyful quality of life worth living. A whole being is connected and aligned and, when out of alignment, knows how to get back into alignment. You either want more out of life or you want less out of life!

The media and institutions are clever with the words they choose to use to get you to do what they wish: Consume until you are broke or broken. It becomes obvious when you start thinking about the things that matter to you, your family, and your community. You begin the process of thinking about your personal responsibility and this empowers your purpose in life. It all begins with the words *you* choose to use and how *you* choose to interpret the words used toward you. Consider the cleverly chosen slogan "the war on cancer." Every time these words are used, they elicit an emotional response in the minds and attitudes of the American people. The word *war* means *fighting*. This so-called "war" began in the early 70s as the "fight" for the cancer "cure," and we have been "fighting" ever since, with our money. In fact, we are "fighting" all these diseases that "plague" our society while also being taught we are fragile beings that can only sit and wait until a disease "attacks" us.

What are we taught to do in response? We do whatever the corporations that designed this system tell us to do, even though it always seems to involve harmful, legalized, FDA-approved drugs, harmful surgeries, and harmful tests. We are taught to "fight" back with our money and time, but not with common sense. What we obviously need is more legalized, FDA-approved drugs, surgeries, treatment plans, and early detection machinery cleverly called "prevention." Right? One popular magazine recently said we need new "weapons" against disease.

These words are so important because they elicit emotional chemical reactions that create physical responses that drive our neurological systems and condition them. If you hear something often enough, you begin to believe it and even defend it. This is why the American population is currently wired to "fight" with emotion rather than common sense. Again, this is due to programming that blames disease on everything outside the body—and now people even blame their own genes. Clever, no? Think about it. Every time you go to the doctor's office, you fill out an intake form and family history. The family history reinforces the idea that your emotional and physical health is connected to other family members who share your DNA, and this plants the seed in your thoughts. You will be amazed and liberated, once you step outside this collective social consciousness, how easy it is to see the truth. Just think of all the magazines and major media outlets that, year after year, boast about a possible "cure" in a new pill or new treatment program that never comes to fruition. Well, it never will because you can never "cure" the physical body from sickness, disease, deterioration, degeneration, deformity, or premature death using an outside approach.

Remove all obstructions and allow the body to be normal. A human being must be looked at as a whole being, and the individual must first take back his or her responsibility to self and stop blaming some invisible, fictional bad guy—you know, germs, genes, or whatever is being sold to the public to increase legalized, FDA-approved drug and treatment sales. You can improve your physical body simply by removing limited belief systems and taking physical action steps that will yield a limitless supply of emotional and physical energy.

Fear controls people and paralyzes their ability to think on their own, to receive answers to live by, and to create a life of fulfillment from connection. You are greater than you can ever imagine, and have the power of Universal Consciousness, God, Universal Intelligence, or whatever you wish to call it. With that, you must understand the universal *pure principles* needed to transform and annul your thoughts associated with germs, genes, or whatever they want to sell you this month. If you believe anything, at a minimum believe you are being sold something through fear, and that you are a victim as a result. The only thing you should fear is your own ignorance by not elevating yourself through the power of the spoken word.

- I know I am!

- I know I am not sick!

- I know I am not poor!

- I know I am not weak!

- I know I am healthy emotionally!

- I know I am healthy physically!

- I know I am!

Now you know the power of words. Now you see and hear the difference with how words are used. Just look at how the written words here contrast: I hope I am. I hope I am healthy. I pray I am. I pray I am healthy emotionally. I think I am. I think I am healthy physically vs. I *know* I am! I *know* I am healthy emotionally and physically! See the difference? Now *know the difference* and use it wisely; it is God's multiplication so the word brings forth abundance, and abundance is everywhere. Word is law! It is as simple as that! Declare it, and it will come to pass!

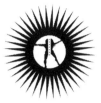

Chapter 5

What Health Is Not— Don't Be Fooled by Sick Care Disguised as "Health Care"

"We don't have a health care system; we have a blood-test-labeling and symptom-treatment system that believes only in FDA-approved, legalized drugs, surgeries, radiation, and harsh testing protocols!"
—Dr. Joey Amato, DC

"We become healthy as well as wealthy by being wise."
—Dr. David R. Hawkins, MD, PhD

A major recurring theme of this book is responsibility to self, which begins the process of awakening to the simplicity of life. Emotional and physical health is simple, yet interactions with others are not always simple. If you understand the universal laws that govern everything and choose to work within these laws rather than against them, you will experience greater control of your life. Do you have more faith in humankind's thousands of years of human-made education or in the billions or trillions of years of the Universal Innate

Intelligence's expression of life in all living organisms? Humankind theorizes and guesses while the Universal Innate Intelligence knows.

What is sold as "health care" in America is both funny and disturbing. The words that are used to sell "health care" in America are also both funny and disturbing. And, while not funny, the negative results of "treatment" plans affecting the quality of millions of lives in America today for profit are, indeed, disturbing. Profits outweigh the risks. Even more disturbing is that America, in a recent study, was ranked dead last for the quality of health and health care against sixteen other affluent nations. America, with only 5% of the total world population, has the largest "health care" system in the world and consumes the largest amount of legalized, FDA-approved prescription drugs. This should be enough to raise an eyebrow and begin the process of asking some quality questions to receive quality answers.

Take a moment to reread the previous paragraph and think about it logically. Every pharmaceutical corporation outside the United States sells the vast majority of its stock to America and keeps only a small percentage for their own country. Logically, we should all be asking why this is so. What is more, America spends the largest amount of taxpayer money on research and development for the consumption of legalized, FDA-approved medications and for surgical procedures, radiation, and harsh testing protocols. America also spends the most amount of money for what is commonly referred to as "health" insurance. Unfortunately, so-called "health" insurance is really sickness and disease treatment insurance based on blood values and other testing protocols always involving large dosages of harmful legalized drugs and radiation.

Let's review. At present, America: 1) has the highest rate of every disease and ailment affecting all people from infants to the elderly, 2) consumes the most legalized, FDA-approved pharmaceutical-"grade" medications, 3) spends the most money on research and development looking for "cures" by way of legal, FDA-approved drugs, surgeries, and harsh testing protocols, and 4) spends the most money per person through what we call "health" insurance. If that is not enough to make your skin crawl, understand this: The leading cause of bankruptcy in America is people's inability to pay for extremely expensive, allopathic medical procedures and legalized, FDA-approved medications when their "health" insurance company stops paying. (Fact: The majority of people who have gone bankrupt have had both a college education and "health" insurance.)

In the years the United States has been under allopathic medical influence, we have had the largest number of diseases ever recorded in the history of humankind. Remember, at present, America ranks number one in incidents of virtually every health-related malady known to humankind (see Chapter 3). Common sense through observation and a few simple mathematic calculations clearly demonstrate that it is simply impossible for America to have epidemics of these proportions resulting from germs, bacteria, viruses, genes, or whatever is being sold this week to scare the living responsibility out of you. Nor is it logical or rational that God the Creator just does not like Americans or the immigrants who come seeking a better life. Common sense observations lead us to conclude that the root cause of the problem is the allopathic medical "health care" system itself.

Equally disturbing is the amount of misinformation produced by the media to elicit negative emotions and opinions that prevent the American people from having the discussions that "We the people" need to start having. Opinions are not facts. Using common sense, it is obvious to me that what separates people in issues of health and "health care" is the identification people have with words and the use of words that create their opinions and their identity. A friend once told me that everyone is entitled to his or her own opinion but not everyone is entitled to his or her own facts. Facts are facts, and what you choose to do with a fact is your decision. The difference between having a superior quality of life and a life filled with sickness, disease, deterioration, degeneration, deformity, or premature death is being able to see through the daily rhetoric that is sold through the media as facts. The language that is used, specifically in allopathic "health care," is what divides people. If people cannot understand or identify with the language being used, they are ignorant to what is truly being discussed and then sold. You pay for it one way or another.

We can easily understand that if we were to travel to another country and did not speak the language we would be at a disadvantage. This disadvantage would be costly if we did not understand it and deal with it ahead of time to ensure we take proper measures for our emotional, physical, and financial safety. This simple analogy easily demonstrates how the use of words, when inappropriate, incorrect, or misunderstood, often leads to emotional, physical, and financial harm, especially as it relates to the topic of "health care." Real, productive, preventative measures begin with knowing the difference and using common sense.

It is easy to see how sickness is a business—that is all it is. If, after a hard day's work, you decide to spend time sitting in front of what my mother called the *idiot box* (television), you will be subjected to massive amounts of rhetoric, useless information, opinions, and lies. Therefore, it is most important to *know the difference* and to use common sense to decipher what is marketing hype and what is entertainment. I daresay most of what you watch on television is marketing and designed to alter your thoughts and opinions, even in the programs that seem to deal with "real life," everyday drama we relate to emotionally. Think of all those in-between advertisements that sell you emotions through words and images of happy, "healthy" people on legal, FDA-approved pharmaceutical grade drugs. Think about the magic pills and potions that are solicited all year long to you and your children. The media sells the idea to the American people, and the idea then becomes woven into the fabric of society. While the emotional and physical effects of all this on the American population is not positive, it is obvious that the institutions involved certainly benefit financially.

The pharmaceutical corporations are among those that, financially, have record-breaking quarters year after year, decade after decade. Advertising corporations know how to sell emotion and belief systems, and they, too, break financial records each quarter, year after year, decade after decade. Look at how well they sell children useless products that damage them emotionally and physically over time and affect their future thought processes, attitudes, and belief systems.

Do you really believe these institutions care about your emotional and physical health or the emotional and physical development of your children? What these institutions want is not only your money but also your devotion and loyalty to their brand. They want you and your family as repeat customers for as long as you all live. While it may be good business, that does not make it right. If what we have covered in the previous pages is the truth—which it is—we have a serious problem that requires immediate attention, as it affects our lives and the lives of those we love.

It is not only a matter of life or death; it is a matter of the quality of life we have in between life and death. How many family members have to suffer? How many children have to continue to suffer at the hands of an ill-informed, misguided parent who clings to legalized, FDA approved pharmaceutical drugs and a system that has failed, and continues to fail us? How many children have to suffer with identities associated with sickness, disease, deterioration, degeneration, and deformity, along with all the negative feelings associated with being diagnosed from blood tests as if something was wrong with them? If left alone, children are born healthy. They have the potential to be healthy. When all interferences are removed they can heal if, in fact, there is an actual problem or situation. Daily, we, as a society, are force-fed information that says sickness is part of our lives and that it leads to diseases that have crippling effects on us as we age. Most parents in America blindly believe in the opinion of another regarding the emotional and physical well-being of their own child or children. We are trained as a society to not question these institutions and those taught by them. Is this normal behavior for a living organism that was blessed with free will or for a mature, well-informed adult?

How do you learn if you do not question? How do you grow if you do not question? How do you change for the greater good? Question everything, especially in regard to your health and the lives of your children. People ask more questions when buying a car than when being diagnosed. They ask more questions when purchasing a computer than when putting something in their own body that is human-made. People ask more questions when purchasing luxury items than when their children are being "treated" either before or after birth. We must all take this situation seriously. Every day that goes by, a child or adult that is subluxated (interfered with) moves closer to sickness, disease, deterioration, degeneration, deformity, and premature death. The business of the constant rhetoric of sickness and the blind faith people have in the institutions that promote sickness is the deadly combination that manifests the results we see today. The fact is, this deadly combination influences the language people use in regard to their emotional and physical health and that of their children, grandparents, parents, uncles, aunts, and anyone moving toward retirement.

People give rhetorical excuses when disease is diagnosed at a later stage of life, specifically, "that it comes with age." This is as ridiculous as people speaking with authority when they receive a diagnosis, or when they say they have the "best of the best" medical specialist. Why is it that everyone claims to always have the best? A person's diagnosis becomes part of his or her identity, as does their allopathic medical doctor. I have never heard anyone say the doctor they are using is mediocre, have you? It certainly makes you wonder why an allopathic medical doctor's malpractice insurance is so ridiculously high.

We often hear people speak of their doctor as follows: "Oh, he is the best because he studied at so and so, and teaches at so and so, and is the head of so and so department at so and so hospital!" or "She is the best because she takes care of all the so and so of that major league team, and she is the head of the department for research and development for so and so disease center at so and so institution!" or "He is just fabulous because he is the head of research for such and such conditions and has done over fifty thousand of these procedures with the highest success rate in so and so city or so and so state!" It is interesting to note that everyone who has the "best of the best" doctor in the "best of the best" specialty hospital or allopathic medical facility, does so in order to feel emotionally secure about their present diagnosis or situation.

Whether it relates to themselves or their child, spouse, parent, grandparent, uncle or aunt, people convince themselves to see what they believe they need to see instead of seeing the truth. At moments requiring this kind of security, the right words are more important than ever. You never hear someone talk without authority; they have to have hope, given the fact they are not in control. They have given up their authority (i.e., their personal power) to someone or to a group they think knows better about what the perceived problem(s) is.

In addition to everything covered to this point, America is also number one in terms of misdiagnoses and malpractice law suits, as well as lawsuits against pharmaceutical drug injuries, known as *iatrogenic effects* (side effects). More often than not, when a person is seriously injured or dies due to side effects from legalized, FDA-approved medications or surgery, it is blamed on the diagnosis/condition and not the system. Some would consider this a great business model, and it is; the problem, however, is that people's lives are at stake. When someone dies or is dying, or is crippled and told to rely on a certain pill or liquid for the rest of his or her life, and the physical body begins to deteriorate over time, the saddest part of not *knowing the difference* is that it is always blamed on the diagnosis which gets added to the national statistics for diseases and death rates. This identification with sickness misaligns and disconnects us from our responsibility to take real action, and this form of fear paralyzes people emotionally and deteriorates them physically over time. Deterioration is never understood to occur as a direct result from subluxations from blood toxicity, tissue toxicity, and cellular toxicity that obstruct the nervous system's innate intelligence to heal normally.

The body heals naturally when provided the right conditions, just as a baby, through natural processes, develops cellularly in a woman's womb. No man, educated or not, can duplicate what comes naturally from the inner wisdom of the innate intelligence within human beings. No matter what the nightly news says, scientists can never get it right, for they neither know nor understand the secrets to life. Life is to be appreciated and supported, not interfered with by guesses, theories, and experiments; it is that simple. Our present allopathic medical "health care" system operates from its own set of theories, guesses, and guidelines that are used systematically and mathematically in very much the same way as the twentieth-century invention of the assembly line which transformed the nation and brought forth the industrial revolution.

This was the beginning of the new age of big banks, big institutions, big industry, and huge, obscene profits, as well as monopolies that arose through various subsidiaries of these primary institutions. This is called *capitalism*, and it is great for business, but not great for the emotional and physical health of "We the people." These capitalist systems rely on their own language (use of words) that the average or outside individual may not comprehend, thus rendering that person at a disadvantage that directly affects his or her thought process, attitude, and belief system.

We already know that medical terminology with its own scary language revolves around the study of sickness, disease, deterioration, degeneration, deformity, and premature death. Why do we not, instead, study life, living, longevity, purpose, power, and action, as these are the very things that make, give, and promote emotional, physical, and financial security? Is there anyone out there who wants to be sick, diseased, physically deformed, or die before their time? I did not think so—I know I certainly do not. That is why allopathic medical terminology is scary and has a negative effect on our thought processes, attitudes, and belief systems. No one wants such a diagnosis or to be on legal, FDA-approved pharmaceutical drugs for the rest of his or her life. No one wants to have repeated surgeries or medical test after medical test.

The language we and others use determines the path we follow: a path that takes us to either a quality of life worth living or a life of sickness, disease, deterioration, degeneration, deformity, and premature death. In Proverbs 18:20, the Bible states: "Death and life are in the power of the tongue, and they that love it shall eat the fruit thereof." This means, of course, that how we use and interpret spoken words determines the world in which we live. What is more, those that love life, and use the power of words to that end, shall reap the most benefit from it.

The opposite also holds true. As touched on earlier, just watch the nightly news and see and hear the negative rhetoric that influences people with doubts of a positive future. If you are hopeless, then you are powerless and can be easily led in a negative direction. The bottom line: You have the power to decide how to interpret what you hear.

Albert Einstein said, "Insanity is doing the same thing over and over again and expecting different results." The causes of sickness and disease in allopathic medicine are always theorized and discussed, but never understood logically. Simply put, we have been "fighting" diseases with massive amounts of tax money and political support for decades, but their "scientists" do not know any more today than they did a century ago. That equates to a hundred years of unchanged thought processes, attitudes, and belief systems that clearly do not work. What Einstein did not realize was that billions of dollars are made annually now, and institutions from Wall Street to Your Street rely on this money exchange. This system is based on a scary language that separates the physician from the patient, putting the ill-informed patient at the mercy of the physician's best guesses.

In college and subsequently in their internship, allopathic medical doctors are taught how to diagnose based on blood values, harsh testing protocols, and their best guess. Always in America a diagnosis is followed by a treatment plan using legalized, FDA-approved pharmaceutical drugs, surgery, or radiation that your "health" insurance covers partially. The diagnosis determines the protocol that is used. Does that sound like health care, or does it sound more like treatment care based on blood values, harsh testing protocols, and a doctor's interpretation?

What about side effects? We know all legalized, FDA-approved pharmaceutical drugs have side effects, right? We have seen, read, and heard the direct-to-consumer pharmaceutical advertisements on television, radio, and in magazines that blatantly warn of the side effects, haven't we? All over-the-counter, legalized, FDA-approved drugs and legalized, FDA-approved prescription medications have side effects with the exception of none; this is a well-known, established fact. In addition to side effects resulting from prolonged use of a drug, drug use can also cause immediate side effects, cleverly labeled *allergic reactions*, as though the patient's body is to blame for the negative side effects. Blame is a great business. Side effects lead to more symptoms, which lead to more diagnoses, which lead to more treatment plans using more legalized, FDA-approved drugs. Any logical human being who is in control and *knows the difference* understands this is a cycle of insanity.

The fact that most of our population over the age of sixty is, in fact, on one legalized, FDA-approved pharmaceutical drug or another is a sad testament to society. Our over-seventy "elderly" community is also on many legalized, FDA-approved pharmaceutical drugs, all with harsh side effects. The side effects get blamed on the person's age and their diagnosis. It is a truly remarkable business plan. There is simply no quality of life and, by blaming age, germs, bacterial infections, failing organ systems, viruses, or whatever other disease label is placed on these people, they are put on more legalized, FDA-approved medications and are subjected to surgeries under the thinking it will save their lives. Statistics, however, prove otherwise.

The allopathic medical system is not focused on the nervous system. In fact, the nervous system has been interfered with (paralyzed and subluxated artificially by human-made synthetic chemicals) for years and is therefore unable to do its job correctly to sustain life. These toxins/poisons obstruct the person's innate intelligence (which is their normal nerve transmission) and interfere with life itself. The business model may be perfect, but the health model is not.

41

By now, you should have a better understanding of what health is not. What, then, *is* health? After all, we have so many people in the "health care" industry that talk about health topics from allopathic doctors, to dieticians, to fitness gurus, to nutritionists, to life coaches, to regulatory agencies that claim to use "scientific" data in regard to the nutrition facts found on the back of everything we eat. But they do not talk about what health truly is. When a hundred people were asked what health meant to them, the most common answers included the following: health is how you look and how you feel; health is determined by blood test results or your [allopathic] medical doctor's opinion based on blood test results and symptoms; health is a prostate exam or a mammogram; health is weight loss, dieting, or calorie counting; health is avoidance of carbs, fats, cholesterol-free foods, or gluten; health is vegetarianism; health is an aspirin a day, taking a legally prescribed heart or liver pill, or taking supplements; health is jogging, exercise, weight lifting, or power walking; health is a glass of wine a day or processed organic foods; health is what I learn from my favorite real-life [allopathic] TV doctor dressed in scrubs; health is this, and health is that. Get the point? Given our different upbringings and backgrounds and the massive amount of chaotic information the media feeds us, it is easy to see why we are confused and frustrated and not getting the long-term results desired for a great quality of life. The sad but true fact is that not one thing listed above represents what health truly is; if it did, we would have the best (not the worst) healthcare system in America.

All this confusion makes it easy for people to rely on the blame game. It is disturbing to see how many people believe what they presently do in regard to their health is good for them when the allopathic medical system still labels and diagnoses some of the worst degenerative diseases we know, adding to the growing demand for legalized, FDA-approved pharmaceutical drugs, surgeries, and radiation. A growing number of independent thinkers, however, are emerging out of the chaos of this current way of thinking in America; they want to annul the system with absolute authority and confidence. Truth is truth and, as the saying in the Bible goes, the truth shall set you free. Sadly, most people do not understand the truth; millions of Americans suffer and prematurely die each year because the American population is not being raised to understand the principles presented in this short book—principles that create the right thought process, attitude, and belief system to create the common sense needed to *know the difference* and work with the Genius Within that is governed by an all-knowing, Universal Consciousness. To begin the process of appreciating what is true emotional and physical health is as simple as understanding the principles presented here. In order to appreciate, understand, and change, we must have something with which to compare.

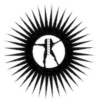

Chapter 6

The Five Components to Absolute Emotional and Physical Health: The Solution

"People who achieve absolute emotional and physical health always do things in a certain way!" —Dr. Joey Amato, DC

"Where there is no vision, the people perish: but he that keepeth the law, happy is he." —Proverbs 29:18

"A man's way of doing things is the direct result of the way he thinks about things." —Wallace D. Wattles, American author

"Seek and ye shall find." Without exception, every problem has a solution; there is no such thing as failure. Failure occurs when you decide to give up the pursuit of achieving a goal. If you make a decision and physically take action to achieve that goal, obstacles will likely show up along the way. That is when you need to *know the difference*, and use your common sense and logic to decide the best way to overcome every obstacle you encounter. Every decision you have made in the past has created your life experiences—both positive and negative—and, as a result, provided you with knowledge. All knowledge, whether from good or bad experiences, is positive. What action steps you take as a consequence of your acquired knowledge is what gives you the potential to manifest into wisdom. Like knowledge, wisdom is also positive.

Wisdom results from your thoughts and beliefs put into action so as to create a positive result for an intended purpose. Your experiences, and how you decide to interpret and act on them, influence your thoughts. Your thoughts, then, through your emotions, influence your actions. The key factors in your thoughts are the words you use to design and create your personal purpose. Daily affirmation toward a clearly defined purpose comes from your ability to decide what you want. The intended outcome of a chosen desire and what you do to fulfill this desire makes the difference. If you hear something enough times, either internally or externally, you will eventually believe it and defend it even if it is a lie that can cause emotional, physical, or financial harm.

The power of repetition creates a habit. Habits will always have either a positive or negative effect on emotional and physical health. A habit that produces positive results is always the result of understanding what you want ahead of time. When you have a clearly defined purpose in life, you will have passion, the fuel that is needed to actively achieve the smaller objectives that must be met in order to fulfill the larger purpose. Passion is the emotional power that creates the drive needed for physical action to take place. Your physical body is the vehicle for carrying out your life's intended ambitions, objectives, and purpose. Therefore, to guarantee ultimate emotional and physical success for the long term, your thoughts and physical body had better be right. What is the use of achieving a goal if you are sick, diseased, deteriorated, degenerated, deformed, or dying prematurely? Emotional and physical health is the one major factor needed for enjoying life's rewards.

It is never enough to hear something of value just once. Positive habits are formed through repetition, consistency, and persistence, all of which develop the necessary momentum for success in any endeavor. Is this not sound advice? Is this not what you would teach your children? The principle of consistency works not only with careers, money, and possessions, but also with the most important factor in human development: emotional and physical health. It is never enough to hear it once.

They say knowledge is power; in fact, knowledge is not power. The *application* of knowledge is power, which means that knowledge, itself, is *potential* power. It is most important to understand that your decisions create both positive and negative experiences. Experience, positive or negative, creates the knowledge that leads to wisdom and helps you to *know the difference* to change future results in your favor.

Life coach Anthony "Tony" Robbins is famous for repeating this insight: "The past does not equal the future." *Knowing the difference* is the wisdom, common sense, and logic needed to ensure emotional and physical stability for the present and for the future. Your acquired experiences, knowledge, and wisdom accumulate in your mind to influence your thoughts, beliefs, and emotions. The right emotions will influence the drive necessary to stimulate you into action—and action gets results.

Repetition of this process and understanding its influence on everything in life creates habits. Whether the habit is healthy or unhealthy depends on your purpose. You must determine and clearly define your personal purpose in advance. What are the emotional and physical results you want? (One always affects the other.) Desire creates passion, passion creates drive, and drive is the energy for action. Simply put, your thoughts and decisions control your physical actions and the outcomes you achieve. Your daily habits determine your attainment of emotional and physical health. Be very selective in the words you use daily and how you respond to the words of others, as this influences and reinforces what will become your habits. No matter how you look at life, if you are a mature adult your emotional and physical health is your responsibility; your health is your number one asset and your number one investment. Once again, who is responsible for your emotional and physical health as well as that of the people relying on you? Consider these choices: a) your allopathic medical doctor, b) your insurance company, c) corporate-sponsored lobbyists, d) your "elected" government officials, e) your spouse, f) your favorite television doctor, g) you. By now, the answer should be obvious.

If you wish to achieve anything in life, you must clearly define the objective you wish to achieve. Everything begins first as a thought which, through imagination, creates the vision to see the end result. If you can visualize the end result, you can make it materialize. A clearly defined purpose is the key factor that, from your emotions, animates the call to action required to materialize what began as a thought. To guarantee success, you must know this ahead of time.

The purpose of the objective for any individual is to first acquire, and then maintain, emotional, physical, and financial health and security throughout life. Remember, nothing is bigger or more important than life. It should be appreciated, respected, and responsibly maintained, as you would maintain any possession held in high regard and value. For, what is the enjoyment or value of acquiring money and possessions without emotional and physical health? What is the quality of relationships with family, friends, loved ones, colleagues, and business associates when you do not have emotional and physical health? What do the most important moments in your life, the so-called turning points, resemble when you do not have emotional and physical health? Imagine going to college, getting married, having a child, purchasing a home—all typical turning points in life—without emotional or physical health. Our defining moments and life experiences as parents, grandparents, sons, daughters, and friends are greatly and negatively affected when there is sickness, disease, deterioration, degeneration, deformity, and premature death. Sometimes, these defining moments called *turning points* do not occur at all.

The first step to absolute emotional and physical health is by changing your thoughts and beliefs. Only *you* can do this for yourself and then for your children. The time has come for people to decide for themselves what is in their own best interest. The days of asking someone else's opinion about your most important asset—your life—are over. Gone are the days of allopathic medicine, theorizing, guessing, speculating, and diagnosing. Gone are the days of "treatment" plans using legalized, FDA-approved harsh drugs, dangerous surgeries, or combinations of these and legalized, FDA-approved harsh testing protocols that lead to more diagnoses that require even more "treatment." Gone are the days of being blindly led by an allopathic medical psychiatrist blindly putting your child on a mental "health" prescription of legalized, FDA-approved drugs or letting someone else dictate to you what is necessary for your child. Gone are the days of being blindly led by an allopathic medical doctor and using over-the-counter, legalized, FDA-approved drugs for every little fever, sniffle, or runny nose. Gone are the days of feeding children nothing but legal, FDA-approved processed chemicals called "food" and blindly believing everything that is written, spoken, or otherwise presented in any form from the media. Gone are the days of saying "I do this because *they say…*" as an explanation to why you do something habitually.

It is ignorant, foolish, and very costly to believe that some person or group has all the answers concerning your emotional and physical health, especially since those answers always involve legalized, FDA-approved drugs, surgeries, and harsh testing protocols. Our current system of allopathic medicine that is governed by "health" insurance has failed "We the people," and it continues to fail. The problem with "health care" in America is not that people do not have access to "health" insurance or are uninsured, as the media portrays; the real problem with "health care" is the "system" itself, and the manner in which it approaches human health, conducts itself, and refuses to change. This "system" of "health care" and its approach is sick, diseased, deteriorated, degenerated, deformed, and dying!

"Change is the law of life. And those who look only to the past or present are certain to miss the future!" —John F. Kennedy

"Our only security is our ability to change!" —John Lilly

"Be the change you want to see in the world!" —Gandhi

"Change your thoughts and you change your world!"
—Norman Vincent Peale

"Our life is what our thoughts make it!" —Marcus Aurelius

"A man is what he thinks about all day long!" —Ralph Waldo Emerson

"Do you want to know who you are? Don't ask. Act! Action will delineate and define you!" —Thomas Jefferson

"Be sure you put your feet in the right place, then stand firm!"
—Abraham Lincoln

"There are three constants in life...
change, choice and principles!" —Stephen Covey

"An army of principles can penetrate where
an army of soldiers cannot!" —Thomas Paine

"To be specific is to exhibit a knowledge of the principles
and art of adjusting!" —Dr. D. D. Palmer, DC

"Principle #32: The Principle of Coordination: Coordination is the
principle of harmonious action of all the parts of an organism, in
fulfilling their offices and purposes!"—Dr. B. J. Palmer, DC

"By adopting the principles you learn from this book,
you can be one of those much-needed achievers!"
—Dr. Sid Williams, DC, Lasting Purpose

Understanding the Law of Maintenance and Using its Principles

"If you can't explain it to a six year old, you don't understand
it yourself." —Albert Einstein

"Life is really simple, but we insist on making
it complicated." —Confucius

"Simplicity is the ultimate sophistication." —Leonardo da Vinci

"A child of five could understand this. Send someone to fetch
a child of five." —Groucho Marx

"There is no greatness where there is not simplicity,
goodness, and truth." —Leo Tolstoy

The Law of Maintenance and its principles are very simple to understand and apply. Its application is the key factor to achieving ultimate emotional, physical, and financial success in life. Do not be fooled or ignorant of the simplicity of this system; too much of our present way of life is overly complicated and leads to confusion. Confusion, of course, leads to frustration, worry, and dissatisfaction, all factors that affect the success of any and all endeavors. If your thoughts and way of thinking are not right, you will fail. Unknowingly, this self-sabotage brings about fear, which then disconnects, misaligns, contracts, subluxates, and shrinks you mentally, emotionally, physically, and drains you financially.

Maintenance of any kind is always affordable and always preserves the integrity and value of what is being maintained; that is what counts. We teach our children to take care of their possessions and to clean their room daily so as to instill values, principles, and the respect of cleanliness and money to ensure the development of great habits. Is this not the definition of maintenance? We teach children the healthy habit of brushing their teeth multiple times a day. Is this not maintenance? We maintain our automobiles, motorcycles, and mechanical possessions to preserve their integrity and value to guarantee an appropriate and quality life span. Homeowners regularly maintain their property to ensure curb appeal and value. People maintain their homes by keeping them clean. Think about what a bathroom would look and smell like if you did not perform regular, consistent clean-ups every day! Is this not maintenance? Maintenance about material possessions is taught to us very early in life, yet it is neither taught nor regularly reinforced about our most important possessions: our life and the future quality of that life.

Our number one asset is our life and the present and future quality of that life. We have been taught to invest in everything except our most important asset, which is something we already possess. What will your future look like? What will be the quality of your life in the future? Will you have multiple diagnoses? Will you be legally medicated and suffer with many different side effects that will lead you to more legalized, FDA-approved medications and more side effects? How many legalized, FDA-approved surgeries will you have while on legalized, FDA-approved drugs? How many "treatment" plans will you be on? Will you be deemed legally handicapped? Will you be deemed legally disabled? Will you need a visiting nurse? Will you require a cane, walker, or wheelchair? Will your children have to place you in a nursing home? Will the muscles, ligaments, tendons, and joints of your spine be so distorted, disfigured, and deformed that the hard bone sits directly on your brain stem and causes your spinal cord and nerves to interfere with your brain's ability to send signals neurologically? Will your muscles, ligaments, tendons, and joints be so malnourished that a little thing like getting in and out of bed will be hard to do without discomfort and pain? Will your organs be so deprived of nourishment and nerve supply that they begin to function abnormally? Will you be physically deformed? Will your muscles, ligaments, tendons, and joints atrophy due to lack of use and years of ingesting processed, man-made chemicals sold as "food"?

How will you age? How will your child or children develop? Who is responsible for the development of their habits? Will your mind and body become sick, diseased, deteriorated, degenerated, deformed, or prematurely die because you did not maintain it regularly? Consistent maintenance of mind and body is the ultimate key factor that guarantees absolute emotional and physical health. "Health" insurance will never pay for maintenance; that is a fact. It will only pay for "medical necessity" based on an allopathic medical doctor's "diagnosis" that has been derived from harsh testing protocols leading to "treatment" plans. This revolving door guarantees one thing and one thing only: a steady stream of money and repeat customers for the allopathic medical system.

Allopathic medicine "treats." It only knows how to "treat." The current "system" is designed to "treat," not maintain. The five components that will be presented in this book are what will guarantee success and is appropriately called principled health care; it is all about maintenance!

Many financial advisors currently design and set up retirement plans for their clients that include money not only for retirement, but also for legalized, FDA-approved prescription drugs, surgeries, visiting nurses, and nursing home facilities. Is this what you envision when you choose to retire? Many retirees spend most of their time visiting allopathic medical doctors instead of enjoying the fruits of their labor. Instead of seeing the world, they are dying prematurely and paying for it financially. The leading cause of bankruptcy in America today is due to costly "health care" payments. Do you believe you are covered? The truth is, you are not. Forget about the fact that "health" insurance focuses only on sickness, disease, deterioration, degeneration, deformity, medical necessity, diagnoses, and "treatment" plans using only legalized, FDA-approved drugs, surgical procedures, and harsh testing protocols and the equipment used, all of which guarantee more of the same. The fact is, "health" insurance has so many loopholes, co-payments, and deductibles that the above-average household goes bankrupt because of this "system."

You move toward the things on which you focus. You must change your thoughts, attitudes, and beliefs. Think about this: Do you want to live and have a quality life, or do you want to live in fear? Fear makes you give up the authority over yourself and those that rely on you. Do you want yourself, or those that rely on you, placed on harsh "treatment" plans with side effects, or do you want to live and have the quality of life you were born to have? What about the quality of life of your children? Do you want to be absolute in your authority in making the right decisions? When you are well informed, you can make the right decisions. Absolute authority comes from being consistent; and consistency gets results, something that guarantees success in life. What does your allopathic medical doctor look like? Does he or she look like the model of near-perfect health? Is he or she physically deformed and out of shape? What are his or her beliefs, focuses, and attitudes? It all matters! You are your #1 investment, so start investing today to maintain your #1 asset: You! You are either growing or you are shrinking, and if you are shrinking you are prematurely dying.

The Five Components to Absolute Emotional and Physical Health

Component #1: Thoughts and Beliefs
Mind Purpose: Mental Maintenance through Daily Affirmation

There is one mental-emotional component to absolute health, Thoughts and Beliefs (Component #1), and four physical components: Spinal Alignment (Component #2), Functional Massage (Component #3), Functional Activity (Component #4), and Body Nourishment (Component #5). The mind is the key factor for each of the five components. Maintain your mental health by focusing on life, living, longevity, purpose, power, and action. Everything begins with a thought. Remember:

- *Knowing the difference* is the key factor.

- Use common sense through observance.

- Use logic.

- Trust the Genius Within.

- Be flexible in mind.

- Adapt to change.

- Know the power of words.

- "The tongue is mightier than the sword."

- Words are extensions of thoughts.

- Words elicit chemical reactions in the physical body.

- Words affect the physical body.

- Words are either positive or negative and create either positive or negative emotions.

Your emotional health directly affects your physical health just as physical health directly affects your emotional health. Your nervous system is affected daily by the choice of words you use, so be selective in your choice of words. Keep the following affirmations in mind throughout the day:

- I am fit, lean, and trim!

- I am great!

- I am successful!

- I am absolute!

- I am emotionally and physically healthy!

- I am an asset and my #1 investment!

- I am!

- I invest in myself daily!

- I invest in my child and my children daily!

- I invest in maintenance!

- Failure is not an option!

Again, since the nervous system is affected by words, be very selective in how you choose to use words as well as interpret the words directed to you each day. The right thoughts and beliefs support rest, relaxation, and adequate sleep, all of which are attributes to health. Do not surround yourself with negative influences when you have a choice to not yield to them.

- Clearly define your purpose!

- Desire things and clearly define your desires!

- Clearly define your overall objective as well as your smaller objectives!

- Take physical action and know that your physical body is a vehicle to carry out your chosen life's ambitions!

- Be ambitious and consistent every day!

- Rest every week!

- Repetition creates habits and habits are either negative or positive!

- Habits can destroy or create!

- Consistency and repetition create confidence!

- Confidence creates sex appeal and sex appeal is desirable!

- Be creative and use your imagination!

- Visualize and desire what you want!

- Never lack in vision and only tell people who will support your vision!

- Never lose imagination or fail to be creative!

- Always be appreciative of your life!

- Always be grateful for the rewards as well as the obstacles!

- Being grateful always inspires!

- Inspiration creates immediate exponential growth!

- Inspiration is emotional fuel!

- This is *passion*!

- This is *power*!

The right emotion creates drive, and drive is the energy needed for activity. Also, drive creates the persistence needed to create success, so never give up your pursuit to happiness. Because you are either prematurely dying or you are living, you are either shrinking or you are growing, you are either decreasing or you are increasing, you are either inflexible or you are flexible, or you are either wanting or not wanting more in life, you must focus on your purpose, use your power, and take action. You and your life are important, and how you choose to live your life is important. You matter first and foremost!

You must accept that you are aging and there is no such thing as anti-aging; nothing prevents aging, but how you age is your choice and that is what matters. The quality of your life matters and depends on your choices and the habits you have created throughout your life. How you choose to live is most important since you will die someday, and how you die is important. Also, it is important to accept the truths in life, but doing something with these truths is more important.

- Accept physical death and live life.

- Focus on life, living, and longevity.

- The legacy you leave behind matters.

- How you raise your children matters because their lives matter.

- How you speak to your children matters.

- Their lives matter.

Your thoughts and beliefs become your observable habits, and your habits create your children's habits. Remember, you are responsible for *you*, and you are responsible for *your children.*

Follow these recommendations:

- Give over 75% of your daily attention to superior things and nothing else.

- Do not focus on things only as they are at present; rather, focus on how you want them to be, and then take action.

- In your daily conversation, speak only of things that add value and allow you to receive value.

- Never blame.

- Ask quality questions so that you receive quality answers.

- Be a leader, not a follower.

- Be absolute.

- *Know the difference.*

In order to understand and appreciate anything in life, you must have something with which to compare. Life is about experiences and the decisions you make based on those experiences. Wisdom comes from life's experiences, and wisdom is *knowing the difference* and being able to direct future events in your favor.

Other considerations:

- Surround yourself only with like minds.

- Focus on life, living, longevity, purpose, power, and action.

- Pay for only what adds value to your life long term.

- Invest financially in you first.

- Invest financially in your child or children's habits now.

- You are your #1 investment.

- Show patience for the results.

- Never give up the pursuit of an intended goal, because failure only happens when you give up the pursuit, and failure is not an option.

- Be flexible in mind and be flexible in spine.

Following all of these guidelines and doing more daily is what creates absolute authority. When you have absolute authority, you can use fear to your advantage rather than be controlled by it. Adherence to these tenets each and every day is what creates absolute emotional and physical health for life. Start investing today, for this is the only way to health!

Component #1: Thoughts and Beliefs
Mental Maintenance through Daily Affirmation

‡ *Failure Is Not an Option* ‡

Component #2: Spinal Alignment
Body Action: Spinal Maintenance through Physical Application

The foundation of the physical body's ability to perform all physical activities is the spine. The foundation of the physical body's ability to function is the spine. There is nothing you do physically that does not involve the spine. Additionally, the spine is the key factor for the four physical attributes of the five components: Spinal Alignment (#2), Functional Massage (#3), Functional Activity (#4), and Body Nourishment (#5). The spine is made from hard bone, which is the hardest substance found in the human body, and is the most overlooked area in human health and development. Physical health directly affects emotional health, just as emotional health directly affects physical health.

The Importance of the Spine

The spine and the skull protect the brain, spinal cord, and the exiting nerves; and the brain, spinal cord, and a portion of the exiting nerves are the only organs that are completely encased in hard bone and protected by it. The brain and the spinal cord are the most important organ structures found in the physical body. The brain, spinal cord, and all nerves in the body comprise the nervous system, and the nervous system controls and coordinates all the functions of the physical body. How well a living organism functions determines its level of health. Therefore, the brain and the spinal cord are the most important organ structures found in the human body; they are vital to human health and development.

Common sense and logic dictate that this area of the body requires special attention and regular maintenance, since the most important factor in physical health is the spine's ability to function the way it was designed to function. By design, the spine is segmented into twenty-four individual and interdependent vertebrae for flexibility, stability, and mobility. If the spine is not flexible, it is not stable, and mobility will always be compromised. Inherently, the spine has four curves that allow the body to maintain weight equally for balance, coordination, and stability, which are the key factors for physical activity and action. The physical body is designed to be fit, lean, and trim so as to disperse its weight evenly to support the spine. The stability of the four curves of the spine supports strength, speed, and stamina. The brain, through the spinal cord, which is supported and protected by the spine, coordinates these physical attributes. Through constant use and repetition, one's strength, speed, and stamina as well as any perfected skill will develop over time. The physical body is the physical vehicle to carry out our thoughts to first survive, then thrive.

- Everything begins with a thought.

- The structure determines the function.

- The physical body must be maintained in order for it to function correctly and to be of any useful value.

- For the physical body and nervous system to be of any useful value, regular maintenance of the spine is very important.

- The spine is the key factor for all the physical attributes involved in the five components, and regular maintenance of the spine is involved in components #2 through #5, with emphasis on spinal alignment for flexibility.

- Regular maintenance of the spine guarantees your maximum enjoyment, maximum benefit, and maximum life span, thus maintaining the quality and value of your life.

- Regular physical maintenance is a necessary part of our responsibility to ourselves and to those who require guidance, such as children.

Remember, anything that is used daily requires regular maintenance. The spine is used daily, even while we sleep. There is never a moment in the course of the day (or night) that the spine is not used. Life's emotional and physical demands cause the segments of the spine, the vertebrae, to misalign, or subluxate. Life's demands affect muscles, ligaments, tendons, joints, and organs that subluxate the spine. Life's demands affect the nervous system which, in turn, affects the chemistry of the physical body, which affects the muscles, ligaments, tendons, joints, and organs that subluxate the spine. Everything is connected and it is foolish to think otherwise.

Subluxations are a communications breakdown in your body. Subluxations are hard bones crushing soft tissue. Subluxations cause neurological interference, which in turn causes the breakdown of brain-to-body and body-to-brain communication. Spinal subluxations are misalignments of the hard bones that protect the brainstem, the spinal cord, and the exiting nerves. Uncorrected subluxations interfere with the nervous system's natural, inherent, and innate ability to coordinate and maintain normal neurology and also to heal when necessary. Uncorrected, over time prolonged subluxations bring about sickness, disease, deterioration, degeneration, deformity, and premature death, eventually destroying the nervous system by destroying its ability to function. Flexibility is key!

Living things that are dying are stiff and uncomfortable, and things that are alive and growing are flexible to adapt to a constantly changing environment. Be flexible in spine, and flexible in mind.

Serious, severe, acute subluxations are a direct result of extreme negative thinking, severe physical traumas, and man-made processed chemicals. Extreme prolonged negative thoughts, acute physical trauma, and man-made processed chemicals negatively affect the muscles, ligaments, tendons, joints, and organs that support the individual segments of the spine. Organ dysfunction affects the nervous system, which affects the spine, and vice versa. Everything is connected and it is foolish to think otherwise. Uncorrected, prolonged subluxations always lead to stiffness and dysfunction, and dysfunction always manifests into symptoms. All symptoms involve subluxations. While not all subluxations begin with symptoms, given enough time, all subluxations will develop into symptoms.

"As the twig is bent, so grows the tree."

Infants, toddlers, children, and teens use and abuse their spines every day. They are very active in the development of their balance, coordination, and stability. This normal development causes them to constantly subluxate their little spines, yet they have no complaints from symptoms. Just because there are no complaints, however, does not mean they are not subluxated and do not require regular maintenance. Flexibility is key! Children and teenagers who lead active lives and are involved in sports subluxate their spines. Additionally, the constant emotional pressures placed on them from mental and physical activity causes subluxations.

Normal life activity and years and years of a lack of maintenance to the spines of children and teenagers result in untold, uncorrected subluxations that develop into stiff muscles, ligaments, tendons, and joints that then must work harder to regulate weight distribution evenly. Over time this pressure manifests structural imbalances that lead to erosion, decay, and deformity of the body's joints. Because of the lack of maintenance to their spines, children and teenagers develop into sick adults with bad physical habits, deformed posture, protruding heads, slumped shoulders, and often a visible hump in the upper back.

Most adults have bad physical habits and live in some form of physical pain and discomfort—primarily symptomatic of dysfunctional muscles, ligaments, tendons, and joints resulting from prolonged, uncorrected subluxations. Symptoms are our body's way of telling us that something needs to be corrected and then maintained so it can stabilize, heal, and grow. When our bodies are physically maxed-out, the spine—as the foundation of the physical body—is always affected. The human body is very intelligent. Our nervous systems always know what to do, when to do it, how to do it, and in what amounts to do it, as long as it is being supported, maintained, and given sufficient time to do whatever is required of it.

Remember the following:

- You cannot blame the occurrence of subluxations on your genes; they are not hereditary.

- Fear and blame are great for business but not for the emotional and physical health of "We the people."

- Subluxations can never be avoided; they are a part of life's emotional and physical demands.

- Prolonged, uncorrected subluxations become severe subluxations that will always be associated with long-term sickness, disease, deterioration, degeneration, and deformity—all leading to premature death.

- You use your spine daily, so maintain it.

- Subluxations also result from stiffness and irritability caused by lack of sleep.

- Tension in and around the neck, mid-back, lower back, and hips are a direct result from subluxations and vice versa.

Subluxations are caused by the following:

- Prolonged negative thoughts and beliefs.

- Negative words that cause aggravation or fear.

- Confusion, if not understood correctly.

- Frustration from confusion and worry from frustration.

- Worry that leads to fear.

- Fear when not understood correctly.

- A diagnosis or multiple diagnoses (no one wants to be diagnosed.)

- Allopathic medical "treatment."

- "Health" insurance-based "treatment" plans. "Health" insurance plans pay only for "treatment"; they do not, nor will they ever, pay for regular maintenance care.

Section 2251.3 of the Medicare guidelines, which sets the standard in America for all "health" insurance policies, states, in red print, the following regarding maintenance therapy: "*Chiropractic maintenance therapy is not medically reasonable or necessary and is not payable under the Medicare program. Maintenance therapy includes services that seek to prevent disease, promote health, and prolong and enhance the quality of life, or maintain or prevent deterioration of a chronic condition.*" What?!? Is this for real? Read it again, and then read it again. Do you fully comprehend the meaning of those specific words? Below we reverse them to drive home the point of what our "system" of allopathic medicine and "health" insurance does, in fact, pay for: "*Allopathic, legalized, FDA-approved medical treatment is medically reasonable and necessary and is payable under the Medicare program. Allopathic, legalized, FDA-approved medical treatment therapies include services that seek to promote disease, promote sickness, and shorten the quality of life, or neglect or assist the further deterioration of a chronic condition."*

This notion runs contrary to the principles of chiropractic founded in 1895 by D. D. Palmer, and then, after his death, further built upon by his son B. J. Palmer. Much later, when chiropractic was "accepted" into "health" insurance, its founding principles were changed and distorted so that a chiropractor could get reimbursed financially. Prior to its "acceptance" by the allopathic medical profession, chiropractic terminology related to life, living, and longevity. In fact, the discovery of chiropractic was a direct result of the "health care" system of the time, as people suffered from side effects from harsh, crude treatment protocols that relied on man-made chemicals, crude surgeries, and best guesses from so-called experts. Times have not changed much, but technology certainly has. Chiropractic focused on services that prevented disease, promoted health, and prolonged and enhanced the quality of a life, and it also maintained and prevented deterioration of chronic conditions caused by malnourishment, factory labor, and the allopathic medical system's approach to "health care." Think about that! Remember, everything is connected and it is foolish to think otherwise.

Think about what we know about allopathic "health care," and "health" insurance:

- "Health" insurance plans do not pay for regular maintenance care.

- You must be labeled (diagnosed) legally handicapped and legally disabled in order to receive what those in the industry call "maintenance," which is, in fact, "treatment," given what it involves.

- Handicapped and disabled people are always subluxated.

- All legalized, FDA-approved medications cause subluxations.

- All legalized, FDA-approved medications taken regularly cause severe subluxations.

- All legalized, FDA-approved surgeries cause severe subluxations.

- All legalized, FDA-approved harsh testing protocols cause severe subluxations.

- All side effects, joint dysfunction, organ dysfunction, sickness, disease, deterioration, degeneration, and deformity involve subluxations.

- All people who die prematurely had severe subluxations.

- Lack of regular spinal alignment (a.k.a. spinal hygiene a.k.a. spinal maintenance a.k.a. spinal adjustments) causes subluxations.

- Lack of regular functional massage (a.k.a. spinal-alignment support massage a.k.a. muscle, ligament, tendon, and joint functional movement massage) causes subluxations.

- Lack of regular functional activity (a.k.a. spinal-alignment support stimulation activities a.k.a. muscle, ligament, tendon, and joint conditioning) causes subluxations.

- Lack of regular body nourishment (a.k.a. spinal-alignment nourishment support a.k.a. whole foods and raw juices a.k.a. intelligent whole foods) causes subluxations.

A lack of regular physical maintenance through the Five Components to absolute emotional and physical health causes restrictions that cause subluxations to your #1 asset, you. Physical health directly affects emotional health, just as emotional health directly affects physical health. Everything is connected and it is foolish to think otherwise.

- Be flexible in mind and in spine, as it will keep you in line.

- You are responsible for your spine, the foundation of your physical body.

- Invest in maintaining your spine.

Component #2: Spinal Alignment
Spinal Maintenance through Physical Application from:
Principled Chiropractors Certified in T5C, a.k.a.:
Principled Spinal Alignment Specialists Certified in T5C

‡ *Failure Is Not an Option* ‡

Component #3: Functional Massage
Body Action: Muscle, Ligament, Tendon, and Joint Restriction Release Through Physical Application

The foundation of the physical body's ability to function and to perform all physical activities is the spine. There is nothing you do physically that does not involve the spine. The spine is the key factor for all the physical attributes involved in the Five Components, specifically the four physical components of spinal alignment (#2), functional massage (#3), functional activity (#4), and body nourishment (#5). Our muscles, ligaments, tendons, and joints support our spine, spinal alignment, spinal function, and the physical body's ability to perform all physical activities. Everything we do involves our muscles, ligaments, tendons, and joints; they are very important physical attributes involved in the Five Components, and they are controlled, coordinated, and regulated by the nervous system. Specifically, the muscles, ligaments, and tendons stabilize and support all twenty-four vertebrae and the four curves of the spine. Common sense and logic dictate that this area of the body requires special attention and regular maintenance.

- Restricted muscles, ligaments, tendons, and joints cause: subluxations; physical immobility leading to the stagnation of blood flow; inflammation; decrease in oxygen, (vital for life); joint disease, deterioration, degeneration, deformity; pain and discomfort; improper weight distribution causing structural imbalances thus affecting function and manifesting into compensations; irritation to nerves not protected by hard bone.

- Restricted muscles, ligaments, tendons, and joints negatively affect: the flow of lymphatic fluid, thereby affecting our body's most important way to get rid of inner cellular waste which, in turn, negatively affects the nervous system.

Remember, everything is connected and it is foolish to think otherwise. The causes of restricted muscles, ligaments, tendons, and joints cannot be avoided; they are a part of life's emotional and physical demands. Uncorrected, prolonged restrictions always lead to stiffness that causes subluxations and dysfunction, manifesting into symptoms and leading to severe restrictions over time. These severe restrictions will always be associated with long-term sickness, disease, deterioration, degeneration, and deformity. Severe restrictions of muscles, ligaments, tendons, and joints are direct results of extreme negative thinking; severe physical traumas, and man-made, legalized, FDA-approved processed chemicals.

Since you use your muscles, ligaments, tendons, and joints daily, you must maintain them. To accomplish this successfully, it is important to know:

- You cannot blame the occurrence of restrictions on your genes; they are not hereditary.

- Handicapped and disabled people are always restricted.

- All legalized, FDA-approved medications cause restrictions, and medications taken regularly cause severe restrictions.

- All legalized, FDA-approved surgeries cause severe restrictions by way of scar tissue.

- All legalized, FDA-approved harsh testing protocols cause severe restrictions.

- All joint and organ dysfunction involves restrictions.

- All sickness, disease, deterioration, degeneration, deformity, and premature death involve restrictions.

- All people who die prematurely had severe restrictions.

Children and teenagers must maintain their muscles, ligaments, tendons, and joints as they develop and mature. Regular maintenance for you and your children is most important for muscles, ligaments, tendons, and joints, to guarantee maximum enjoyment, maximum benefit, and maximum life span thus maintaining the quality and value of life.

- Lack of regular spinal alignment (a.k.a. spinal hygiene a.k.a. spinal maintenance a.k.a. spinal adjustments) causes restrictions which cause subluxations.

- Lack of regular functional massage (a.k.a. spinal-alignment support massage a.k.a. muscle, ligament, tendon, and joint functional movement massage) causes restrictions.

- Lack of regular functional activity (a.k.a. spinal alignment support stimulation activities a.k.a. muscle, ligament, tendon, and joint conditioning) causes restrictions.

- Lack of regular body nourishment (a.k.a. spinal alignment nourishment support a.k.a. whole foods and raw juices a.k.a. intelligent whole foods) causes restrictions.

A lack of regular maintenance through the Five Components to absolute emotional and physical health causes restrictions that cause subluxations to your #1 asset, you. Physical health directly affects emotional health, just as emotional health directly affects physical health. Everything is connected and it is foolish to think otherwise.

- Be flexible in mind and in spine, as it will keep you in line.

- You are responsible for your muscle, ligaments, tendons, and joints.

- Invest in maintaining muscles, ligaments, tendons, and joints that support your spine.

Component #3: Functional Massage
Muscle, Ligament, Tendon, and Joint Restriction Release
Through Physical Application from:
Principled Functional Massage Therapists Certified in T5C

‡ *Failure Is Not an Option* ‡

Component #4: Functional Activity
Body Action: Muscle, Ligament, Tendon, and Joint
Development Through Physical Application
If You Don't Use It, You Lose It!

The foundation of the physical body's ability to function and to perform all physical activities is the spine. There is nothing you do physically that does not involve the spine. The spine is the key factor for all the physical attributes involved in the Five Components, specifically the four physical components of spinal alignment (#2), functional massage (#3), functional activity (#4), and body nourishment (#5). Our muscles, ligaments, tendons, and joints support our spine, spinal alignment, spinal function, and the physical body's ability to perform all physical activities. Everything we do involves our muscles, ligaments, tendons, and joints; they are the physical attributes involved in the Five Components, and they are controlled, coordinated, and regulated by the nervous system. Specifically, the muscles, ligaments, and tendons stabilize and support all twenty-four vertebrae and the four curves of the spine. Common sense and logic dictate that this area of the body requires special attention and regular maintenance.

Functional activity is the intense use of muscles, ligaments, tendons, and joints within a specific intended period of time for the purpose of developing strength, speed, stamina, and coordination. Functional activity is muscle, ligament, tendon, and joint training at its best, and uses the body the way it was intended to be used. It balances the muscles, ligaments, tendons, and joints to ensure the proper weight distribution specific to each person's body type. All people have different body types with unique characteristics and attributes, so functional activity, along with body nourishment, keeps the body fit, lean, and trim, which is the way the human body is supposed to be. Being fit, lean, and trim is a choice.

A fit, lean, and trim body supports waste removal, weight distribution, and spinal flexibility so you have the ability to perform action, which is the physical activity used to carry out intended goals without discomfort or pain. By developing the body's nervous system through stimulation and use, and supporting flexibility in all areas of the body as you age, functional activity creates the right chemistry to support the nervous system and spinal function. Functional activity:

- Guarantees you will age gracefully.

- Is for all ages.

- Guarantees emotional and physical strength.

- At its best, pushes you mentally to your limits and beyond, showing you what you truly are capable of.

- Inspires desire for more.

- Is sexual activity and vice versa.

- Is common sense.

- Guarantees looking great.

- Guarantees confidence and sex appeal.

Our muscles, ligaments, and tendons are designed to be firm, which is neither too tight nor too loose. Handicapped and disabled people are always physically, functionally impaired.

All legalized, FDA-approved medications restrict functional activity, and those taken regularly cause severe restrictions to functional activity.

This is also true for all legalized, FDA-approved surgeries and harsh testing protocols. Joint and organ dysfunction, sickness, disease, deterioration, degeneration, and deformity all involve restrictions that impair functional activity. Regular, frequent functional activities guarantee maximum enjoyment, maximum benefit, and maximum life span, and thus maintain the quality and value of your life.

Healthy habits are formed early in life. One very important habit is to have regular physical functional maintenance for muscles, ligaments, tendons, and joints. Children and teenagers also have muscles, ligaments, tendons, and joints that require regular maintenance and conditioning so they can mature and develop correctly.

- A lack of regular spinal alignment (a.k.a. spinal hygiene a.k.a. spinal maintenance a.k.a. spinal adjustments) causes restrictions which cause subluxations, thereby impairing functional activity.

- A lack of regular functional massage (a.k.a. spinal-support massage a.k.a. muscle, ligament, tendon, and joint functional movement massage) causes restrictions, thereby impairing functional activity.

- A lack of regular functional activity (a.k.a. spinal alignment support stimulation activities a.k.a. muscle, ligament, tendon, and joint conditioning) causes restrictions, thereby impairing functional activity.

- A lack of body nourishment (a.k.a. spinal alignment nourishment support a.k.a. whole foods and raw juices a.k.a. intelligent whole foods) causes restrictions, thereby impairing functional activity.

A lack of regular maintenance through the Five Components to absolute emotional and physical health causes restrictions that cause subluxations that impair the functional activities used by you, your #1 asset. Physical health directly affects emotional health, just as emotional health directly affects physical health. Everything is connected and it is foolish to think otherwise.

- Be flexible in mind and in spine, as it will keep you in line.

- You are responsible for your body's ability to be active so that you may perform functionally great.

- Use it or lose it.

- Invest in functional activities that support your spine.

Component #4: Functional Activity
Muscle, Ligament, Tendon, and Joint Development
Through Physical Application from:

**Principled Personal Functional Training Instructors
Certified in T5C**

**Principled Group Functional Fitness Training Instructors
Certified in T5C,**

**Principled Functional Physical Movement
Instructors Certified in T5C,**

**Principled Functional Foundational Yoga Instructors
Certified in T5C,**

**Principled Mixed Martial Arts Instructors
Certified in T5C**

‡ *Failure Is Not an Option* ‡

Component #5: Body Nourishment
Body Action: Intelligent Body Nourishment
Through Physical Application

The foundation of the physical body's ability to function and to perform all physical activities is the spine. There is nothing you do physically that does not involve the spine. The spine is the key factor for all the physical attributes involved in the Five Components, specifically the four physical components of spinal alignment (#2), functional massage (#3), functional activity (#4), and body nourishment (#5).

Body nourishment supports the spine, spinal alignment, spinal function, and the physical body's ability to perform all physical activities. There is nothing you do physically that does not involve your body's need for fuel. Body nourishment supports all the physical attributes in the Five Components and is controlled coordinated, regulated, and distributed everywhere by the nervous system. Body nourishment nourishes all twenty-four vertebrae of the spine, and stabilizes and supports the four curves of the spine. Given today's FDA-approved, man-made, processed, and chemical-laden world, common sense and logic tell us that nourishing the body requires special attention and focus, including spinal maintenance, functional massage maintenance, and functional activities.

Intelligent Food for Intelligent People

The body is nourished only by intelligent whole foods, which are foods from the land. They include any life form, such as edible plants and animals, taken from their natural environment. Our daily intake every week should be over 80% whole foods from the land. Whole foods include:

- Raw vegetables, raw fruits, raw nuts, and seeds.

- Pasture-fed, free-range animal meat that does not contain hormones or antibiotics.

- Sea, lake, and river life caught fresh from its natural habitat.

- Water.

Whole foods support:

- All the organs, muscles, ligaments, tendons, joints, and cells of the whole physical human body, including the spine and nervous system.

- Spinal alignment; functional massage restriction releases; functional activity; and provide energy, strength, speed, stamina, and coordination.

Pure raw organic juices, a type of whole food, are the key factor in body nourishment for today's fast-paced world. Well over 50% of our daily intake at least five days a week should be raw vegetables and fruits. Pure raw juicing is the absolute best way to receive whole body nourishment. They flush out the FDA-approved, man-made, processed chemicals found in everything cleverly disguised as "food" that cause subluxations, sickness, disease, deterioration, degeneration, deformity, and premature death. Pure raw organic juices:

- Nourish all organs, muscles, ligaments, tendons, joints, and the cells of the physical body, including the spine and the nervous system.

- Nourish and support spinal alignment; functional massage restriction releases; and functional activity to provide energy, strength, speed, stamina, and coordination.

- Nourish, cleanse, and replenish the body immediately upon entering the blood stream.

- Cleanse the whole body.

- Bring about youthful appearance, skin suppleness, skin elasticity, and firmness.

- Keep the body fit, lean, and trim.

- Keep body chemistry balanced.

- Increase oxygen uptake.

- Support the nervous system's ability to use the nourishment they provide to balance and heal any and all conditions.

The nervous system knows what to do, when to do it, how to do it, and in what amounts to do it, as long as it is supported, maintained, and given enough time. You do not need to know what is in an organic, non-processed tomato, raw vegetable, raw fruit, or any whole, raw food to know it is great for you. It is as simple as that! Honestly, if you have to think about what you are eating, you should not be eating it. If you cannot pronounce the words on a "food's" ingredient list or if you spend time reading its so-called nutrition facts, you should not be eating that "food" or feeding it to an unsuspecting child. Remember, everything is connected and it is foolish to think otherwise.

- A lack of regular spinal alignment (a.k.a. spinal hygiene a.k.a. spinal maintenance a.k.a. spinal adjustments) causes restrictions which cause subluxations thereby impairing the use of the nervous system's ability to correctly coordinate the use of nourishment.

- A lack of regular functional massage (a.k.a. spinal-support massage a.k.a. muscle, ligament, tendon, and joint functional movement massage) impairs the use of that which nourishes the body.

- Lack of regular functional activity (a.k.a. spinal alignment support stimulation activities a.k.a. muscle, ligament, tendon, and joint conditioning) causes restrictions, thereby impairing the use of nourishment and effective waste removal.

- A lack of body nourishment (a.k.a. spinal alignment nourishment support a.k.a. whole foods and raw juices a.k.a. intelligent whole foods) causes malnutrition.

A lack of regular maintenance through the Five Components to absolute emotional and physical health causes restrictions that cause subluxations that impair the functional activities used by you, your #1 asset. Physical health directly affects emotional health, just as emotional health directly affects physical health. Everything is connected and it is foolish to think otherwise.

- Be flexible in mind and in spine, as it will keep you in line.

- You are responsible for your body's nourishment.

- Invest in body nourishment for it nourishes your nervous system and your spine.

Component #5: Body Nourishment
Intelligent Cellular Support Through Physical Application from:
Principled Body Nourishment Specialists Certified in T5C

‡ Failure Is Not an Option ‡

In order to understand and appreciate anything in life, you must have something with which to compare, and now you have that. The intention of this book is to expand your present thought process, attitude, and belief system in regard to your emotional and physical health so that you can take action and be responsible. The truths in this book are both absolute and timeless.

The discovery of this new system of health care is a direct result of the needs of our times. This new system is principled in its beliefs, and has a moral code of conduct of right and wrong which influences its actions. It is based on universal truths seen through the observance of the world around us and is simple to apply and understand. This new, organized system is rightfully called Principled Healthcare.

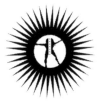

Declaration of Emancipation: My Resolutions

- I do solemnly resolve, before myself, to take absolute responsibility for my emotional and physical health and the emotional and physical health of those that rely on me, such as my child or my children.

- I will no longer give up the authority that I inherently possess over myself and others who rely on me in areas such as emotional, physical, and financial health.

- I will use common sense and logic in gathering facts to make informed decisions in all areas of my life, especially with my emotional and physical health because, without these two attributes to life, my life will become substandard and this I do not accept.

- I will annul sickness, disease, deterioration, degeneration, deformity, and premature death, for I now possess enough knowledge to know that these things are within my control and depend on the decisions I choose to make.

- I will take time to read things of a superior nature so as to add value to my life and that I may add value to the lives of others.

- I will concentrate and focus my thoughts and beliefs on life, living, longevity, purpose, power, and action.

- I will make time for myself first, knowing that this is not selfish, for if I am not emotionally, physically, and financially healthy, I am of no use to others that rely on me.

- I will make time for appreciation, for there is always enough time to appreciate both the obstacles and the rewards in life. I know that being grateful inspires me to be great, and this creates my vision to do great things.

- I will no longer cast blame, play victim, make excuses, or rationalize for the things in my life that I do not like. Instead, I will see the role I play in the movie of my life and take action to grow and change, for my life is within my control.

- I will be selective in choosing how I use words daily, for I now understand their true power.

- I will be selective in choosing how to interpret words directed toward me daily through conversation and through the media, for I now understand the true power of words.

- I will clearly define my purpose.

- I will be creative, and use my imagination to visualize what I want ahead of time in regard to my emotional and physical health, for these are my most valuable assets.

- I will invest in me.

- I will invest in those that rely on me.

- I will take action.

- I understand and agree that people who achieve absolute emotional and physical health always do things in a certain way.

- I understand and agree with the logic behind the Five Components to absolute emotional and physical health.

- I understand and agree with the concepts and principles of maintenance over "treatment."

- I understand that my "health" insurance does not cover maintenance, because maintenance seeks to prevent disease, promote health, and prolong and enhance the quality of my life.

- I declare and understand fully that I am not being "treated" for any condition, label, or diagnosis, and I choose to take full responsibility for the maintenance of my body over any form of "treatment."

- I understand and appreciate that I am the key factor for the success of my life.

- I understand and appreciate the unique process and language used daily at Westchester Life, for it sets a standard of efficiency and results that guarantees success.

- I understand that maintenance involves the services of other like-minded individuals that are qualified and certified in the Five Components to Principled Healthcare.

- I understand and agree with the policies and procedures of Westchester Life.

- I understand and agree that, in order for me to be successful emotionally, physically, and financially, I must read *The Absolute Truth and Common Sense*, written by Dr. Joey Amato, DC.

- I understand and agree that no human being or group of human beings such as a corporation or governing body is responsible for my emotional, physical, or financial health.

- I understand and agree that, in order to achieve ultimate, absolute success, I must create great habits.

- I understand and agree that a necessary attribute to absolute success is being consistent.

- I understand and agree that I am my #1 asset and my #1 investment.

- I choose to be a client not a "patient."

- I choose to be a client at Westchester Life because, as a client, my thoughts matter, my input matters, and my actions matter.

- I choose life, living, longevity, purpose, power, and action over sickness, disease, deterioration, degeneration, deformity, and premature death.

- I choose life, living, longevity, purpose, power, and action over "health" insurance-based medical necessity which is only determined by an allopathic medical diagnosis that always involves "treatment" from legalized, FDA-approved medications; legalized, FDA-approved surgeries; and legalized, FDA-approved harsh testing protocols.

- I choose to seek services that prevent disease, promote health, and prolong and enhance the quality of my life.

- I choose to do things in a certain way to ensure ultimate, absolute success emotionally, physically, and financially.

I AM

I AM FIT!

I AM LEAN!

I AM TRIM!

I AM GREAT!

I AM SUCCESSFUL!

I AM ABSOLUTE!

I AM EMOTIONALLY HEALTHY!

I AM PHYSICALLY HEALTHY!

I AM AN ASSET!

I AM MY # 1 INVESTMENT!

I AM REPONSIBLE!

In order to understand and appreciate anything in life, you must have something with which to compare. Life is about our experiences. Life is about the decisions you make based on those experiences. Nothing is larger than life. Wisdom comes from life's experiences.

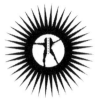

Acknowledgments

I am appreciative, grateful, and inspired by:

Giuseppe Legend Amato

Viviana Love Amato

Daniela Amato

Mom

Pop

Aunt Teresa

Uncle Tony Martino

Dominick Acquista

Rick Caccavale

Gaetano Lombardo

Tony Celentano

Daria Amato

Justine Amato

Joey Vastola

Chris Amato

Pasqual Pelosi

My uncles

My aunts

My cousins

My nieces

My nephews

My friends

My adversaries

LIFE UNIVERSITY

Dr. D. D. Palmer, DC

Dr. B. J. Palmer, DC

Dr. Sid Williams, DC

Wallace D. Wattles

Napoleon Hill

Morris A. Bealle

Ernest Holmes

Albert Schweitzer

Dr. David R. Hawkins, MD PhD

John F. Kennedy

Martin Luther King, Jr.

John Lilly

Gandhi

Norman Vincent Peale

Marcus Aurelius

Ralph Waldo Emerson

Thomas Jefferson

Abraham Lincoln

Thomas Paine

Albert Einstein

Confucius

Leonardo da Vinci

Leo Tolstoy

Lao Tzu

Sun Tzu

Andrew Carnegie

Dale Carnegie

Og Mandino

Anthony Robbins

Paulo Coelho

Gregg Braden

Stephen R. Covey

John Lennon

Bob Marley

Abraham Maslow

Masaru Emoto

Dr. Carolyn Dean

Dr. Pasquale Cerasoli, DC

Dr. Jim Sigafoose, DC

Dr. D. D. Humber, DC

Dr. Reggie Gold, DC

Dr. Fred H. Barge, DC

Dr. John F. Demartini, DC

Dr. Patrick Gentempo, DC

Dr. Thurman Fleet, DC

Eckhart Tolle

Dr. Rob Schiffman

Dr. Ben Lerner, DC

Dr. Thomas O. Morgan, DC

Dr. Ray Omid, DC

Dr. Roger Sahoury, DC

Dr. Chris Zaino, DC

Dr. Tedd Koren, DC

Michael E. Gerber

Christopher Hitchenson

Robert Greene

Steven Pressfield

Paul Zane Pizer

Dr. Arno Burnier, DC

Richard Bandler

John Lavalle

Dr. Bronner

Paul C. Bragg, ND

Patricia Bragg, ND

Dr. N. W. Walker

David Wolfe

Dr. Gabriel Cousens

Dr. Fred Bischi

Gary M. Null, PhD

Dr. Joseph Mercola

Dr. Len Horowitz

Mike Adams, Health Ranger

Dr. Max Gerson

Barbara Loe Fisher

Dr. Bob Hoffman, DC

Dr. John Reizer, DC

Rick Sapio

Dr. Dennis Perman, DC

Dr. William P. Mckenna, DC

Dr. Jonathan S. Zimbardo, DC

Craig Yellin

Jeff Hays Films

The Citizens Commission on
  Human Rights (CCHR)

Rave Diet

Nick Mussolini

Pat Mussolini

Kris Defilippi

Vincenzo Carrini

Carl Ulzheimer

Dominick DeLuccia

Primo Rossetti Jr.

Louis Gasparre

Romeo Spiniello

Dr. David Dick, DC

Dr. Wendy Dick, DC

John Castagnini

Joey Labosco

Dr. Wayne Dyer

Louise L. Hay

Gregg Braden

Joshua Rosenthal

Rick Sapio

THE BOOK

Stephanie J. Beavers

Ghislain Viau

TEAM ELITE

Tonya Dimarco

Emil Paolucci

Maurice Johnson

Eric Berger

Jamie Harris

Greg Watson

Vennesa Cesareo

MARKETING TEAM

Matthew T. Trummer

Maiker A. Cabrera

Dayanara Mercado

Grayson Bevil

Joseph Alvarez

Lindsey TJ Hall

Joseph Salpietro

THE LOFT NYC 2003-2013

Lisa Collarossi, RIP

Yasmin Insanalli, LMT

Lisa Scalere

Dr. Bronstein, DC

Dr. Federico Gonzalez, DC

CWA 1101

MUSIC

MAD SEASON

TOOL

MASSIVE ATTACK

Clint Mansell

Nick Cave & Warren Ellis

Hans Zimmer

Luciano Pavarotti

Frank Sinatra

Dean Martin

BODY NOURISHMENT ESTABLISHMENTS

Mrs. Green's

WHOLE FOODS MARKET

TRADER JOE'S

New York Establishments:

PURE FOOD AND DRINK

BAREBURGER

JUICE PRESS

LIQUITERIA

ORGANIC AVENUE

QUINTESSENCE

PURE FOOD AND WINE

RAW SOUL

LEARNING INSTITUTIONS & SEMINARS

Dynamic Essentials

New Beginnings

Palmer College of Chiropractic

Dr. Max Gerson Institute

Institute of Integrative Nutrition

Anthony Robbins Foundation

Demartini Institute

Chiro Transform

Chiro Business Finishing School

Lululemon Retreats

FUNCTIONAL ACTIVITY TRAINING

CrossFit

Boxing

MMA Training

Krav Maga

Sports Performance Training

Corrective Exercise Training

Jiu jitsu

Martial Arts

National Strength and
    Conditioning Association

National Athletic Trainers
    Association

International Kettle Bell and
    Fitness Federation

Beachbody

P90X

Insanity

TRX Suspension Training

Yoga

Yogahaven

Yogaworks

Dahn Yoga

SoulCycle

Spinning

Pilates

Cardio

Boot camps

Hard Bodies Extreme Fitness, NY

Superhuman Group Fitness, NY

Contenders Club Fitness, NY

Athletic Sports

Soccer

Baseball

Hockey

Football

Basketball

Rugby

Softball

Gymnastics

Squash

Track and field

Tennis

Lacrosse

Swimming

Water polo

Skiing

Snow Boarding

Mountain bike riding

Cycling

Jogging

Golf

Volleyball

Cricket

CRU

Hiking

Equestrian Riding

Ice Skating

Dancing

Ballet

Cheerleading

TOP TRAINING FACILITIES

Equinox

Club Fit

Saw Mill Club, Mount
    Kisco, NY

New York Sports Club

Premier Athletic Club,
    Montrose, NY

Healthy fit, Mamaroneck, NY

Bodyfit, Scarsdale, NY

Extreme Fitness, Mount
    Vernon, NY

Lifetime Athletic, Harrison, NY

Kinetic sports club, Pelham, NY

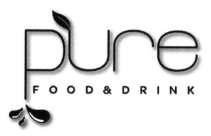

The 5th Component
Body Nourishment

The body is nourished only by intelligent whole foods, which are foods from the land.

They include any life form, such as edible plants and animals, taken from their natural environment.

Pure raw organic juices, a type of whole food, are the key factor in body nourishment for today's fast-paced world.

Fit, lean, and trim is the new sexy!

www.purefoodanddrink.com
914 771 PURE

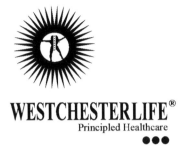

WESTCHESTERLIFE®
Principled Healthcare

●●●

Call Today and Make a Reservation for What We Call The Experience!

Your reservation at Westchester Life, a quality-of-life corporation, is called The Experience because it is just that. The time is now for you to be responsible for your emotional and physical health. The Experience will explain and clarify how to go about achieving absolute emotional, physical, and financial success. Remember, everything is connected and it is foolish to think otherwise! Stop wasting time, energy, and finances seeking "treatment"-based plans, and come experience The Experience for yourself. Visit our website and call or email us today!

www.westchesterlife.org
914-713-8515

Come experience what life has to offer at Westchester Life:
A quality-of-life corporation
Failure is not an option!
You either want more or you want less!
You are your #1 investment!